SYSTEMA
SOLO TRAINING

Robert Poyton

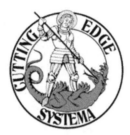

Published by Cutting Edge

ISBN: 978-0-9956454-3-1

DEDICATIONS

With respect and gratitude to Mikhail Ryabko,
and Vladimir and Valerie Vasiliev
for their generosity and guidance.

Thanks to Gareth Ashby, Ed Phillips,
Andrew Chapell-Lewis, Matt Kaye and everyone else
who helped in the production of this book.

Special thanks to Lara Poyton for her photography
and continued patience and support.

ABOUT THE AUTHOR

Robert was born in the early 1960's in East London.
He trained in Judo and boxing as a child and at age
18 began training in Yang Family Taijiquan.

For many years he studied the Chinese Internal Arts in depth.
In the 1990's he set up his own school and began cross
training in several styles.

Robert trained with Vladimir Vasiliev on his first visit to the UK
in 2001 and has trained at Vladimir's Toronto school
several times. He has also travelled to Moscow for intensive
training with Mikhail Ryabko and his senior instructors.
In addition he has arranged numerous UK seminars for
Mikhail, Vladimir and other leading instructors.

Robert now trains solely in Systema and was one
of the first registered UK instructors.

He has been featured in martial arts books and magazines
numerous times as well as publishing his own magazines.

Outside of training Robert is a professional musician
and currently lives in rural Bedfordshire with his wife
and several chickens.

*"Rob Poyton has been training and teaching Systema
since 2000. He is a dedicated and talented instructor,
knowledgeable on all of the key components of Systema.
Rob presents his teaching in a clear and structured
manner through his classes and reading materials."*
- Vladimir Vasiliev, October 2019

CONTENTS

CHAPTER ONE: INTRODUCTION
How to Use This Book 10
How Often to Train? 11
What Equipment? 12

CHAPTER TWO: BASICS
Relaxation 15
Form 16
Movement 17
Breathing 17
Core Exercises............................ 19

CHAPTER THREE: MOBILITY
Joint Mobility 24
Ground Mobility 27
Movement Chains 33
Walking & Running 34

CHAPTER FOUR: STRETCHING
Leg Stretching 39
Body Stretching 42
Moving Stretches............................ 46

CHAPTER FIVE: EQUIPMENT
The Stick 49
The Chain 54
The Hammer 56
Weapons 61
The Environment......................... 74

CHAPTER SIX: HEALTH
Massage 79
Diet 84
Mindset 87
Energy Work 90

CHAPTER SEVEN: PROGRESSION
Progression 95

CHAPTER EIGHT: CONCLUSIONS
Conclusions 102

CHAPTER ONE

INTRODUCTION

*"A wise man is full of strength,
and a man of knowledge
enhances his might."*
- Proverbs 24:5

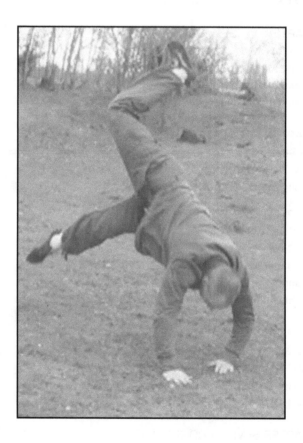

SOLO TRAINING

There is a long tradition of solo training in Oriental martial art styles. Many of these arts have long, involved routines (kata or form) encompassing the style's particular techniques and movement methods. They form a major part of training and are what most people visualise when you say "martial arts".

Russian martial arts developed along different lines. Even in the older forms of sword work there are no lengthy kata, as far as I have seen. There may be some specific movement patterns, but they are typically practiced in a free-style way. Indeed my experience has been that the vast majority of Systema training involves two or more people.

This means that solo training may be downplayed - but it is an important part of our development. Body and mind must be as capable as possible of carrying out the work and solo training is an excellent way of achieving this. It is also very useful, of course, for training at home, or those times when training partners are not available.

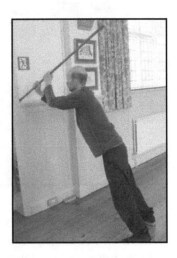

Given that there are no kata in Systema, people often look to exercises for their solo training. This is by no means wrong, but there are many other aspects of work that can be developed on your own.

Our aim with this book is to give you a range of solo training methods. On the face of it, this may seem straightforward - everyone knows about push ups, squats, etc, right? Well, perhaps, but there two important principles underlying any type of Systema training.

The first is that the exercise is not harmful to the body or psyche - it builds rather than destroys.

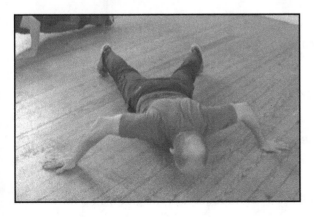

The second is that the exercise feeds directly into the functional aspects of training. Nothing should be done for show, or for the sake of it. Attributes from solo training should be directly mapped onto practical work. As a quick guide to this concept, think on how push ups on the knuckles relate

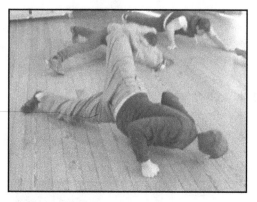

exercise. Always start at a place of comfort before challenging yourself further. We rarely recommend working to failure and always advise you bear safety in mind.

The aim of solo training is to strengthen yourself physically and psychologically in order to support to your daily activities, be they training, work or leisure. The benefits of good exercise are wide and varied and have a profound effect on your well-being. How important, it is then, to ensure your training regime is fit for purpose.

to certain types of striking work. Or how, when you drop your weight in order to throw or takedown a person, you are actually doing a squat. Think how ground mobility exercises play a major role in ground fighting. The reverse is also true, you may find particular movements or techniques that can be revered engineered as solo exercises

How you train depends on your circumstances. Solo training can help with particular goals or activities you are involved in, or just be part of a

There are a huge variety of exercises that can be done and even the most basic exercises can be adapted, changed and tweaked in many ways. There is no way that a single book could cover every type of stretch, every variation of push up and so on, so we have restricted ourselves here to covering the basic types of exercise in each category. But we will also give you some guidelines and a useful framework for developing exercises further.

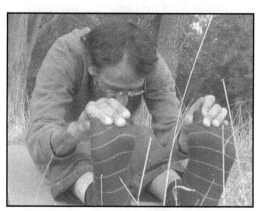

general "wellness" plan. Look for balance in everything, don't be lazy but don't become obsessive either.

HOW TO USE THIS BOOK

A final word before we start - if you have any existing or suspected medical condition, always check with your healthcare professional before undergoing any new fitness regime or

The aim of this book is to give you an introductory overview of Systema solo training. It is by no means exhaustive but will give you a firm foundation in the main areas of training. You can use this book to add exercises to an existing routine, or you can use it to structure and develop new routines and methods.

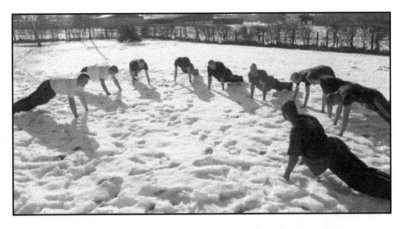

If you are an Instructor or run a training group we hope this book will also give you some ideas for classes. With a little imagination you can adapt many of these exercises for pairs or more. Some can even form the basis of training drills (see our other book *The Ten Points of Sparring* for more ideas).

Although the title of the book is Solo Training there is nothing to stop you using the exercises for a group or class. In fact, every class should contain some element of exercise in it, I feel. If nothing else, it is very good preparation for the work to come. Working in a group also tends to motivate us a little more, it is less easy to give up then when you are training with others!

In our *Systema Partner Training* book we look at how many of these exercises can be adapted to be practiced in pairs, threes, or even larger groups - but it it best to master the solo versions first. We also hope that you will use the ideas here as a springboard from which to develop your own exercises. Creativity is an important aspect of Systema training and it is good if you can develop beyond the norm and keep things fresh and challenging.

HOW OFTEN SHOULD I TRAIN?

This depends very much on your circumstances, time/space available, physical condition, etc. I like to train

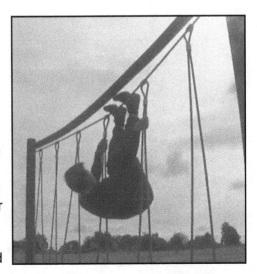

every day. That will typically cover breathing, stretching and mobility work along with some strength training. I tend to do at least one exercise round with the stick daily and of course we should try and monitor our breathing, tension and posture as often as we can throughout the day.

If you don't have much free time, try breaking your training down into ten minute chunks. Even that is enough to do the core exercises a good few times. It doesn't take long to do a few stretches - and in some ways it is better to do them as we need them, rather than wait for our "training time". If you can take this approach you will find you can be training almost all the time - remember the world is our gym!

The important thing is to be consistent. It is better to do 15 minutes a day than nothing all week, then an hour on Sunday. Consistency brings small, but sustained, growth. There are no shortcuts!

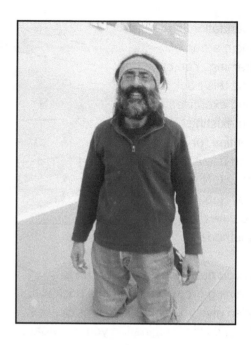

WHAT EQUIPMENT DO I NEED?

There is very little specialised equipment required for solo training and nothing in the way of "gym machinery". The single best piece of equipment you can get is a simple stick. It should be about 4' long and thick enough to bear your weight. I've found a cut -down curtain pole or similar to be ideal.

Other items include a length of chain, some balls of various sizes (tennis up to medicine ball) and any type of weapon (we recommend a training version at first).

If you can fit one somewhere, a pull-up bar is a good

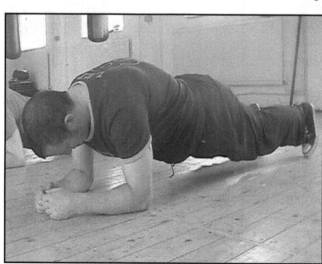

investment. If you want to try weights then look at getting a sledgehammer or kettlebells.

As we just mentioned, it is good to get into the mindset of *the world is our gym*. This means seeing the potential in anything as a piece of exercise equipment. A chair can be used to elevate the feet for press-ups. You can try lifting it from the floor by one leg. You can climb on and around it, or dive over it.

Even just being outdoors gives us a huge range of things to work with, including uneven terrain to run or roll over, trees to climb, getting used to being being cold or hot and

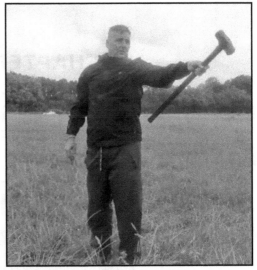

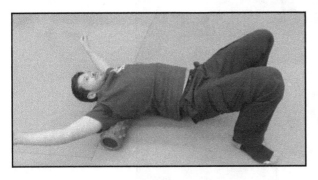

perhaps most importantly renewing our sense of connection to the natural world around us. How much more revitalising than being in a sterile gym environment!

What clothing your wear for training also depends largely on circumstances. As a general rule something loose and comfortable is good. But is is also useful getting used to working in thick winter clothing, heavy boots, or just even your regular

day wear. This also helps the process of exercise becoming an natural part of you rather than it being a "special time"

Of course we always bear safety in mind and, if we are to take risks, at least to be aware of and prepared for the consequences.

Finally the most important piece of equipment is your brain! Approach solo training with joy and creativity, not the desire to punish yourself. See difficult movements as a challenge, if necessary break your work down into stages.

Be as consistent as you can, the greatest progress comes through small but regular steps. Even with illness and injury you can work some aspect of physical / psychological training.

In short - don't give up, always keep moving!

CHAPTER TWO
BASICS

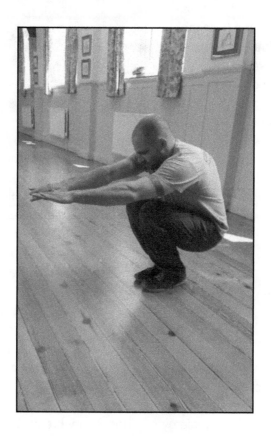

BASICS

There are certain principles that are fundamental requirements of Systema training and should be present in all activities. Whether engaging in solo or group training, we should always be mindful of these requirements.

THE FOUR PILLARS

Systema is often said to be built on four major principles - the Four Pillars. They are relaxation, form, movement and breathing. The practitioner should understand the role of each in any type of exercise or drill. We will briefly look at the first three principles in turn, then take a more in-depth look at breathing, as it is the most important of all.

Although we often separate them for ease of learning, we should remember that in reality there is constant inter-action between all of these principles. We should also bear in mind that there is a psychological as well as physical aspect to each principle too.

RELAXATION

In our activities we are looking to accomplish any given task with just the required amount of tension. If we look at fitness training in general it is not uncommon to see people doing fast squats with red faces and hunched up shoulders. People get the pulse elevated and so feel they are achieving something. Unfortunately all

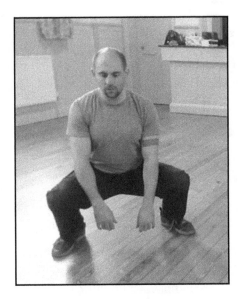

they are often doing is increasing the tension within the body with a corresponding risk to health.

For the most part we are seeking to perform any exercise or movement with the minimal amount of tension. For a push-up this means relaxing the shoulders, holding the body straight and keeping just enough tension in the hands and wrists to maintain the structure - think of the body as a bridge, it has to be strong in the right places, but if the whole structure is tense and immovable it will fail under load.

Some exercises call for us to tense muscles - either specific muscles or the whole body. The purpose of these exercises is usually to help us release accumulated tension, or in order to help strengthen a particular part of the body. As we will see later, Systema stretching is built heavily on the idea of releasing tension rather than "stretching the muscle". We try and avoid moving under tension - or at least

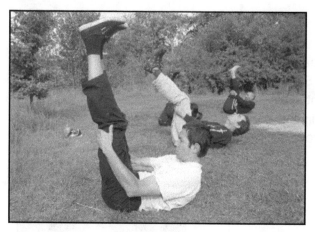

moving fast. Slow movement under tension can be useful for some things, but should always be done with care.

Try to get in the habit during the day of regularly "checking yourself" for unwanted stress. Over time you will get a feeling for controlling your tension and how to get rid of any excess. This in itself is one of the greatest benefits of solo training, as stress is a leading cause of numerous modern lifestyle ailments.

FORM

By form we mean good posture and practical knowledge of your body on a bio-mechanical level. As unwanted tension is released, you will find ways of using or organising your body structure with greater efficiency. To return to our push-up example, you will find that with correct form you are able to "rest on the bones" rather than use tense muscles to support your body weight. Exactly the same principle applies to standing or sitting.

Achieving this in static posture is one thing, doing so in solo movement is another. Adding in pressure from outside in form of a partner or equipment adds in another level of challenge.

If you want to get a feel for good basic posture, simply stand upright and relax the body, without slouching. Imagine you are holding a stick across your shoulders (or actually use a stick, see later chapter). Your shoulders and hips should be level, it is surprising how many people carry one side higher than the other. Check in a mirror or have someone correct you. Your head should not lean or jut forward. To get this feeling, place your hand on the crown of your head, grab some hair (if you have some!) and pull lightly upwards. You should feel the neck stretch slightly and the chin tuck in a little. This is the optimum position for the head. The spine too should be straight, with no lean or kinks. Think of the spine as an antenna, with the head atop. The better its shape, the more information it can take in and relay.

There are many resources available to learn about bio-mechanics and also many new developments going on in sports science. It is good to get a sound scientific understanding of how the body operates - as well , of course, as corresponding information on psychology and the like. However intellectual understanding is always a support to physical work and can never replace "body knowledge".

MOVEMENT

With relaxation and good posture comes free movement. Through correct exercise we can explore our range of motion, develop strength in different vectors ,improve how we walk, run, climb and so on. I feel that freedom of body movement also brings with it a sense of liberation. It is hard to be "uptight" when the body is free and relaxed. This takes us back to a time when we were children - watch how young kids move, often with very little tension and no preconceived notions or mental blockages.

The notion of "playfulness" is an important and powerful aspect of solo training. Even the most challenging exercises should be approached with a focused but playful mindset rather than the "no pain no gain", suffering mindset. Pain is inevitable, suffering is an option!

BREATHING

No type of Systema training should be undertaken without at least a basic understanding of breathing. We advise that you consult the many resources available from Systema HQ that go into greater detail, but here are some of basic methods to use when training.

Unless otherwise directed, the procedure is to inhale through the nose and exhale through the mouth. People typically exhale upon exertion, which is fine, but is is also good to get used to inhaling on exertion too. Breathing should be comfortable, not over filling or completely emptying, unless otherwise directed. Learn to breathe smoothly and to the requirements of the situation.

When you first start out it is advisable to practice breathing in a safe and comfortable position. If you have any blood pressure or other health issues, always check with your healthcare professional prior to training.

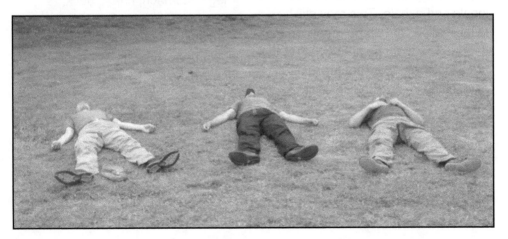

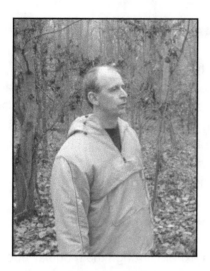

DEPTH OF BREATHING

There are three main "depths" of breathing. The first is shallow or *burst breathing*. Think of a dog panting, the breath comes in the nose and straight out of the mouth. This is most often used as a recovery breath, or in stressful situations. So if your system is stressed you can use burst breathing to regain control and return to a state of equilibrium

The second is our normal, everyday chest breathing. The ribcage expands and contracts with each inhale and exhale. This may still be fairly shallow, or can be practiced more deeply. The main point to watch is that there is no unnecessary tension, particularly in the shoulders.

The third is abdominal breathing. This is where the diaphragm is fully used in order to draw and expel the breath. This can be "normal", where the diaphragm pushes out on the inhale, in on the exhale, or "reverse breathing" where the diaphragm pulls in and up on the inhale and expands out on the exhale.

We recommend you begin with chest breathing, then burst breathing for recovery. Deeper breathing is best trained under the supervision of a good Instructor. Here are some simple solo exercises to get you started. Remember, check out the material from Systema HQ for more in-depth work. If at any time you feel dizzy, then come out of the exercise immediately and sit quietly to recover.

NORMAL BREATHING WITH TENSE / RELAX

Find a comfortable position, standing, sitting or prone. Inhale nose, exhale mouth for a while, slowing the breathing.

Then on the inhale, tense a body part. Just the one section, the rest of the body stays relaxed. Repeat two or three times. On the exhale, relax the body part. A typical sequence might be – legs, stomach, chest, back, shoulders, arms, head.

To finish, tense and relax the whole body three times on the inhale/exhale

WAVE BREATHING

On the inhale, tense the whole body, starting with the feet up to the crown of the head. The wave of tension matches the speed of the breathing. On the exhale, relax from the crown of the head to the feet. Do this three times then reverse the direction.

BREATH HOLDS AND RECOVERY

Inhale and hold for as long as you can. Do not overfill the lungs, work to about 80% capacity. Try and feel where the tension begins in your body. Work to move it or dissolve it. When you release, use burst breathing to recover. Repeat on an exhale/hold

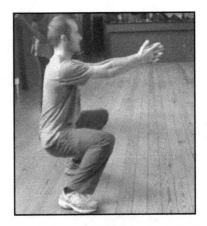

work to keep your breathing smooth and even.

PYRAMID BREATHING

Walk or jog – one step inhale, one step exhale. Gradually increase – 2, 3, 4 etc up to 10. Each time the breath should stretch over the amount of steps. From 10 work back down to 1 again. Take your time and work only up to your limit. Over time, push the limit

SQUARE BREATHING

This follows the same procedure as above, but you add in a breath hold. So inhale 2, hold 2, exhale 2, hold 2 and so on. You can increase the breath hold along with the step, or keep it at a constant number.

These are some basic patterns which we will also add into the various exercises described later. If no particular breathing pattern is described, then the default is to exhale on the exertion or the stretch. Unless directed otherwise, never hold the breath during the exercise and always

CORE EXERCISES

These exercises form the "spine" of solo training. They are designed to work the three areas of the body,upper, middle and legs. They appear simple, but as you progress through your training you will find deeper and deeper levels in these apparently basic movements.

When movements are simple, it is very easy to do them wrong and we tend to just blast out repetitions of the exercise. This is not the Systema approach! Instead, make sure you pay attention to posture, tension and breathing - in other words, the Four Pillars. When you do so, you will find that these simple exercises are actually very challenging to do perfectly.

For this reason it is best to start with slow to moderate speed at first. A good idea is simply to follow the length of your normal breath, with the breath slightly leading the movement. So from the low push-up position, start to exhale, then allow your arms to push the body away from the floor. As the exhale finishes, so does your movement. There are many benefits to his approach, not the least of which is learning how breath can power your movement.

What we will do first is describe the basic version of each exercise. Once you have a reasonable understanding of these, you can go on to try some of the variations.

PUSH UPS

Place the fists under the shoulders. If you find it difficult to work on the knuckles at first, use a soft surface or mat.

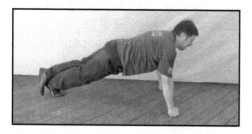

The body should be held straight but relaxed. Ensure that the back does not arch or bow. On an inhale, slowly lower yourself to just above the floor. On an exhale raise the body up.

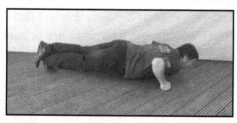

Try not to engage the shoulders, imagine instead you are pushing the floor away. Keep the head looking

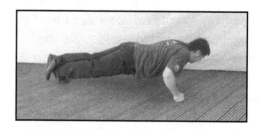

forward, don't let the body sag.

SIT UPS

Lay flat on the floor, inhale. On the exhale sit the body up to 90 degrees. Keep the arms relaxed at the sides and watch for tension in the legs.

Inhale and lay back down again.

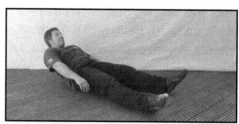

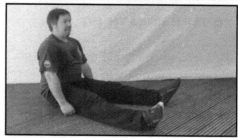

LEG RAISES

The same start position as above. Exhale and slowly raise the feet.

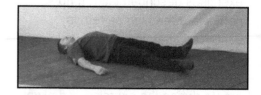

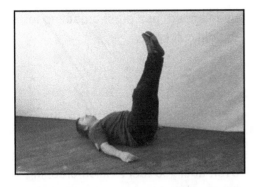

Lift the feet over the head, or as far as you can manage. Once again the body should be relaxed.

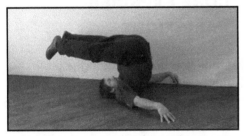

Inhale and return to the start position

SQUATS
Stand with the feet shoulder width apart and parallel.

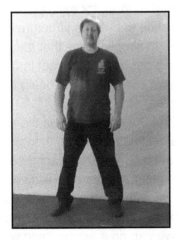

Slowly squat down on the inhale. Try and keep the back straight.

If the feet need to turn out, be sure that the knees remain in line with the toes.

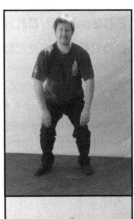

Stand back up on the exhale. Try and keep the back straight throughout.

It is better to go only part way down with a straight back than go full squat with a curved back.

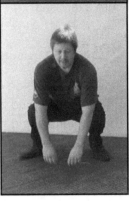

These, then, are the basic exercises which form the foundation of much of our work. If you find them difficult at first, you can do push-ups from the knees, or use a chair or similar to help support yourself during squats. Emphasise form, relaxation and breathing rather than repetitions.

Learn to perform these exercises well and they will prepare your body for much of the work with a partner. Once you can do each one smoothly, then join them together in a continuous flow. So do, say, 15 squats and, on the last one, drop straight into push up position, from there flip over for you sit ups and leg raises. Breathe on the transitions too!

BREATHWORK AND CORE EXERCISES

We can add in various breath patterns with these exercises in order to provide a challenge, enhance our breath control , work on the psyche and so on. Here are some ideas, which can be applied to each of the core exercises

HOLDS

Inhale and hold, do one rep. Exhale. Inhale and hold for two reps. Exhale. Inhale and hold for three and so on, up to five reps. Now work back down to one again. Repeat, but hold on the exhale.

PYRAMID

Try the pyramid breathing pattern with the exercises. So inhale/exhale for one rep. Now inhale one, exhale one. Inhale two reps, exhale two. Go up to five then back down again.

BURST OR SLOW

Burst breath and time the rep with the speed of the breathing. Also practice slow breathing with corresponding slow movement. Also try the reverse, burst breath and move slow, breath slow and move fast.

THE TWENTY COUNT

Do the rep slowly, to a count of 20 (don't rush!). Maintain good form and even speed, use burst breathing for the difficult spots

STATIC

Hold the push-up position (at the top), the squat, sit-up, leg raise (at halfway position). Keep the breathing even until you feel tension creeping in, then go into burst breathing to help dispel the tension.

CORE EXERCISE VARIATIONS

Once you have a good grasp of the basic core exercises it is good to start bringing in variations. There is a simple way to do this, a "formula" we can apply to give us a wide range of practicing the basic movements. That formula is the Four Pillars. Here's how it works - think of each of the pillars in turn and how they can be varied.

If we take Form, for example, we can relate that to the structure of our body. In simple terms that means moving our hands and feet into different positions while doing the exercise.

So for a squat, start in the normal shoulder width position, then move the feet out a bit wider on each squat. Once you have gone as wide as you can, bring the feet all the way back in on each squat until they are touching.

We can do a similar thing with push ups, moving the hands and feet around in different positions. Try

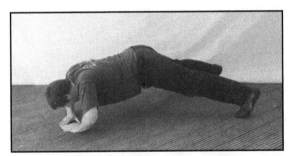

ideas. Start a squat in a relaxed posture, as you go down deeper, add in more tension. So at the bottom of the squat, the body is fully tense. As you rise up, relax in time with the movements so you are fully relaxed at the top of the squat. Of course you can switch this sequence around and use it for the other core exercises too.

starting with the hands under the shoulders, then move them out a little on each push-up, until they are as far apart as you can manage. Then decrease the distance each time until the hands are touching. You can do the

You could also try selective tension during an exercise - just keep one part of the body, say and arm or a leg tense throughout the movement.

Another option is to try and do the exercises totally relaxed, floppy even. For the squat sink all the way to the floor and, from that resting position try and raise yourself with absolute minimal use of muscles.

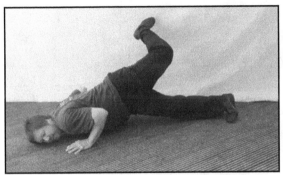

same thing with the feet, of course, or try things like lifting them as you do the push up.

For Movement, think of the speed of the exercise and how you can alter it. Try from very slow to as fast as you can. Try slow on one part of the movement, then fast on the next. You can also hold each exercise as a static position too, or experiment with freezing and holding your posture at different points through the movement.

For Relaxation here are a couple of

These variations are important as, not only do they challenge us in new ways and keep the basics fresh, they also teach us ways to organise our bodies under less than optimal conditions. Imagine, for example, you are injured or exhausted, yet still have to move and function.

Practicing exercise variations will educate your body as to how to work in different ways.

So play around with these variations, I am sure there are others you can find too, particularly once you add equipment or a partner into the mix!

CHAPTER THREE
MOBILITY

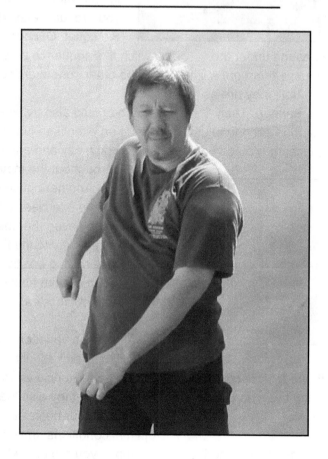

MOBILITY

Mobility is the ability to move ourselves in an efficient and effective way. A way that minimises impact and wear on the body but allows us to complete our task successfully, be it a combat situation or simply walking the dog. A defining factor of Systema is there is no distinction in what you are using your movement for, it is the same process. This is in contrast to a style that may advocate particular stances or specialised / stylised movement for combat situations. Our movement at all times should be natural and free, this way our training truly prepares us for life.

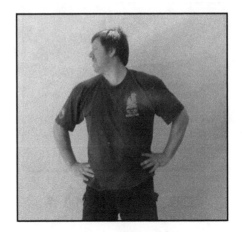

Turn the head slowly to look over the right shoulder, return to the middle, then look over the left shoulder.

JOINT MOBILITY

This exercise sequence is designed to promote a good range of motion in the joints. The movements can be practiced standing or sitting (for the upper body part). Repeat each movement a few times, go slow, keep good form and remember to stay relaxed and breath.

You can run through the whole sequence, or just try one or two during the day to hit a specific problem area. This routine will work all the major body joints, of course there are many variations. You can use this routine as a starting point to explore deeper aspects of joint rotation.

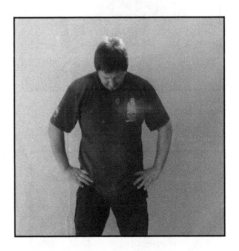

Drop the chin to the chest, bring the head up again, then tilt back and look up. Rotate the head in both directions. Be sure to do this movement slowly and with care, particularly if you have any neck problems. Also keep the shoulders relaxed during this movement.

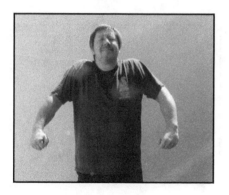

Lift the shoulders as high as
you can on an inhale. Exhale
and let the shoulders drop.

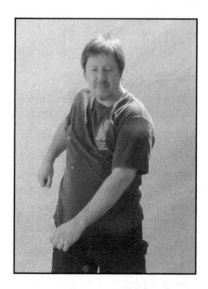

Rotate your shoulders forward,
backward and sideways. Make
as big a circle as you can.

Circle the arms - keep them
straight (but not locked) and
make circles forward, backward
and sideways. Now bend the arms and
circle from the elbows.

Clasp the fingers together
and rotate the wrists.

Inhale and expand the chest,
exhale and let it sink.

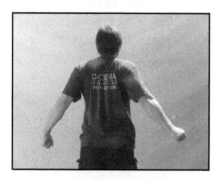

Inhale and squeeze the
shoulder blades back together.

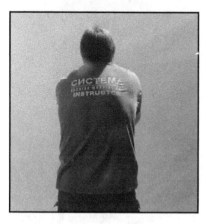

Exhale and open the back out -
imagine you are trying to
touch your shoulders
together at the front.

Keep the
hips and
shoulders as
still as
possible,
move the rib
cage to the
right and left.
Rotate the
rib cage in
both
directions.

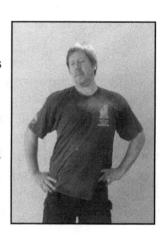

Rotate the hips, be sure to keep the knees relaxed

GROUND MOBILITY

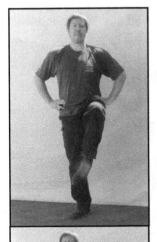

Working from the hip, raise the knee straight up and make outward, then inward circles

Raise the knee and make a forward and backward kicking movement

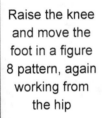

Raise the knee and move the foot in a figure 8 pattern, again working from the hip

Stand on one leg and raise the opposite knee. Rotate the raised ankle, the knee, then the hip. Now change direction and rotate each leg joint again.

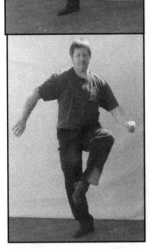

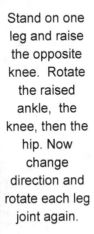

The floor is an excellent training partner - it's always there for one thing! Working on a good surface gives us valuable feedback and forces the body to quickly relax. Of course floor mobility is an essential component of ground fighting but is also a good thing to practice for it's own sake - it takes us back to an earlier age perhaps, when our movements were less inhibited and we enjoyed movement for its own sake.

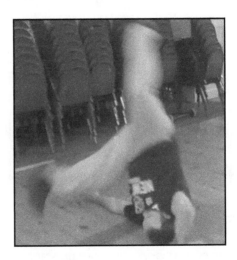

Ground work also teaches us how to manage falling. I often say to people, if you learn nothing else for "self defence", at least learn how to fall! All of us will fall at some stage in our lives, it is a major source of injuries, particularly as we get older. Falling is also excellent for fear control and teaches us a lot about control and acceptance. From a "work" perspective, if we know our partner is skilled at falling, we can work with that much more intensity.

This, then, is a very quick an simple "head to toe" joint rotation routine. Remember, take your time, relax and, above all, breathe!.

ISOLATED FLOOR MOVEMENT

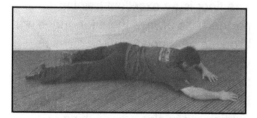

Lay on your back. Use just one part of the body to move yourself around. So you may move by rotating your shoulders, pushing with your legs, dragging yourself with your arms and so on. Work through each body section, then repeat on your front.

SIDEWAYS ROLLING

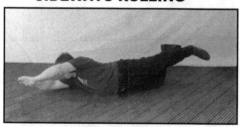

Lay on your back, raise the arms above the head. Raise one knee slightly and thread the other foot through the gap. This will turn your hips and so roll you over. Think of the body as a cylinder.

BACKWARDS FALL

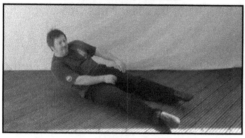

From a sitting position, slowly fall

backward onto the side of the body. Keep the elbows tucked in. Use the momentum of the fall to roll across the shoulders and sit up. Repeat the movement on the opposite side.

BACKWARD ROLL FROM FLOOR

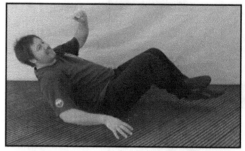

Go into the backwards fall as above.

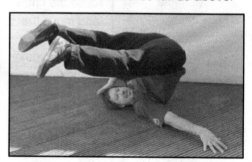

When you fall back, bring the legs over the head, as though you are doing a leg raise. Try this a few times.

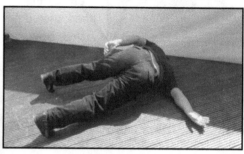

Then, instead of bringing the feet over the head, take them over the shoulder. As the feet get to about 90 degrees, kick out a bit and/or extend your abdomen. This should give you the momentum to roll over the shoulder. Make sure the back of the head does not contact the floor. The arms can go out to the side.

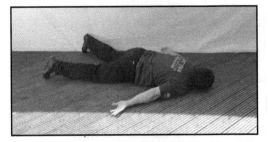

You should end up face down. Exhale on the roll. Go slow at first

FORWARD ROLL FROM FLOOR

From the above position raise your hips from the ground. Push off with your toes and roll over the shoulder.

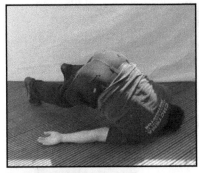

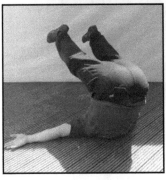

Exhale, go slow, control your speed. You should end up prone on your back.

BACK ROLL FROM SQUAT

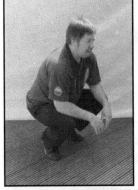

Get into a low squat position. Kick one leg forward and fall back onto your side.

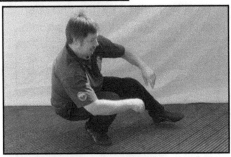

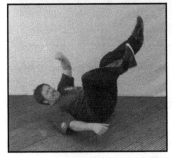

Go into the backward roll as above

FORWARD ROLL FROM KNEELING

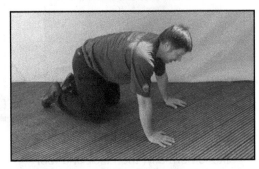

Kneel and place your hands on the floor, to form the corners of a square.

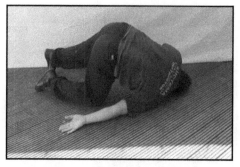

Bring your shoulder to the floor - either sweep the hand across under you, or rotate the hand to the outside. Either way, the shoulder should transition to the floor smoothly.

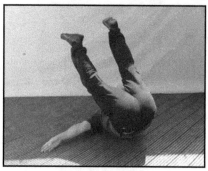

Tuck the head in towards the opposite knee, push off with the feet and roll forward as above.

BACK FALL FROM STANDING

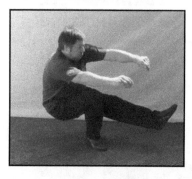

Stand normally, then kick one foot forward and bend the supporting knee (as though doing a pistol squat).

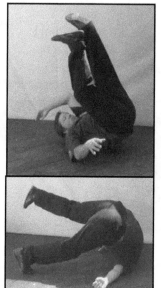

As the side of the buttock contacts the floor, fall back and kick your legs up and over the shoulder, then roll as above.

FORWARD FALL FROM STANDING

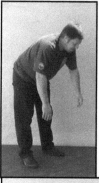

Stand normally, then bend at the waist and take the hands towards the floor.

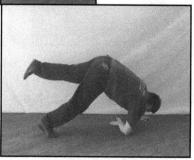

Allow yourself to tip forward and fall.

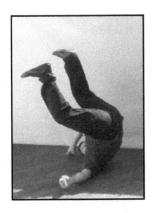

The hand can sweep across under you or rotate to the outside to bring the shoulder smoothly to the ground. Fall and roll as above

Once you are used to this, you can try diving over an object. Try something quite low at first, then build up to the back of a chair.

Take a short run and dive, extending the hands out and also allowing the body to stretch in order to slow yourself down a little. As the hand contacts the floor it acts in the same way as above in order to "guide" the shoulder to the ground. Roll as before.

FORWARD DIVE

Don't go straight into a forward dive, unless you are feeling particularly brave, Instead try this at first!

Find something about waist height that will support your weight and that you can "fall" over. Stand in front of it and push your hips forward. Now slowly lean and let yourself fall, keeping contact with the object.

As you tip forward, bring the hands to the floor and either sweep out or let the arm fold. Remember, never brace! From here go into the forward roll as before.

HANDS AND FEET

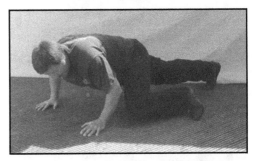

Move around using your hands and feet. No part of the body is allowed to touch the ground. Try working face up and face down.

BODYWALKS

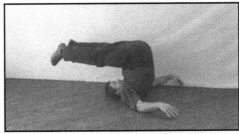

Try "walking" using different parts of the body. From a sitting position, lift your feet off the ground and walk on your butt. Rotate your hips to move! Or get into a leg raise position and walk on the shoulders..

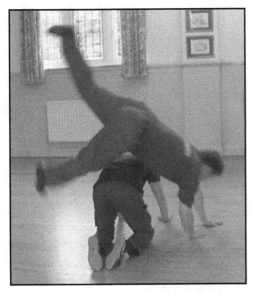

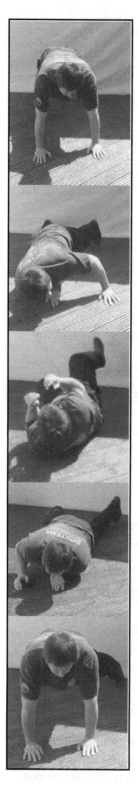

PUSH-UPS FOR ROLLS

If you have problems with the arm rotation for rolls, try this exercise.

Get in push up position on the palms. Rotate one palm inwards in order to bring your shoulder smoothly down to the floor.

Go into a sideways roll and turn until you are face down again.

From here rotate the palm to bring yourself up into the push-up position once more.

The up and down movement should be completely from the arm rotation and not the shoulder muscles.

WORKING FROM THE KNEES

This is a very useful move that we use in a lot in groundwork.

Start in seated position. Tuck your right leg behind you and bring the sole of the left foot to the right knee.

Now swap the leg positions. Twist from the hips to bring the right foot forward and the left leg back

Lift the body and rotate the legs out, so that the right foot is now on the left knee.

Use the momentum of the movement to sit up onto the shins.

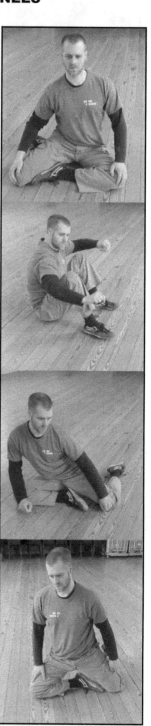

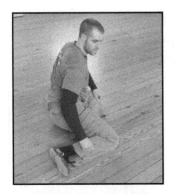

From here you can go back into the original position and begin the sequence over again.

Work first to one direction, then the other. At first it is ok to use your hands for support

MOVEMENT CHAINS

Once you have a reasonable grasp of all the various types of ground movement, start putting them together in "movement chains". What this means is that you do not pause between each move, but flow directly from one to another. This will help in making your ground movement fluid and, through practicing this way, you will also

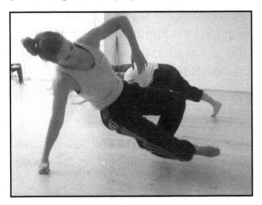

discover "new" movements, or new ways of doing old movements!

You can start with something quite simple, here is an example. From a seated position, go into a back roll, finishing face down. Without pause,

raise the body into push up position and do two of the "push up rolls". On the last one, lower yourself back down and do a forward roll to finish. So that is three movements combined into one "chain". You can easily put together more and, over time, you can aim to be continuously moving for five or ten minutes.

As always, pay attention to breathing and posture and do not rush the movements. If you find there are points where your movement gets a little stuck, or you have to rush through to complete, then repeat that part and try and pinpoint the problem.

For new ideas, routines and movement, take a look at dancers or Play Fight groups, there is increasing exchange between such groups and Systema people.

Once you can move on the floor smoothly, you can increase the challenge by changing your work surface. So if you are using mats at first, try moving on a wooden floor. From here, try grass, concrete, even gravel is possible if you keep the body relaxed. Look around at different places

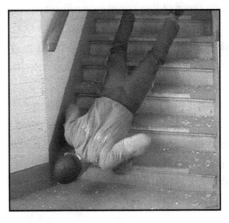

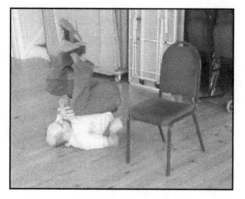

you can work (safely) in, for example try going up and down stairs.

Another layer of challenge is provided by adding objects and obstacles to mover over, around and through. A simple thing is to start with a stick, just lay it on the floor and roll over it in different ways. Use a chair or table and move under, around and over them. You could use a series of obstacles or group them as a kind of ground "assault course".

WALKING AND RUNNING

Walking and running are two exercises that are easy to do and in most cases are very easy to fit into our daily routine. However even these simple things must be done correctly in order to get the most benefit from them.

When running or walking we should always be mindful of our posture and also check for tension, particularly in the shoulders.

It's not uncommon to see joggers with shoulders up around there ears, fists clenched, grimacing. It looks like torture not exercise! I also dread to think about the impact on knees, especially when people run on concrete.

For an efficient running posture, keep the shoulders relaxed, let the arms hang loose at the side, or bend 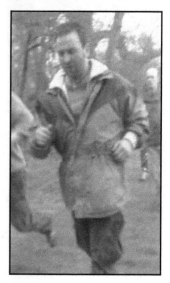 the elbows to bring the hands up to waist level. When you step for running or walking think about how you lift the foot. Try this simple exercise. Lift a foot off the ground, but do it in such a way that the whole foot leaves the ground at the same time - in other words the sole of the foot stays parallel to the floor.

You will find to do this you have to rotate the hip - in other words you use the hip to lift the leg as opposed to engaging the large muscles in the thigh. This is similar to the way you can raise the hands/fists by rotating the shoulders.

Build this method of stepping into your walking / running and you will find there is much less impact on the knees and your steps will be "lighter".

Once posture and tension is sorted, let's move on to breathing. Running is an ideal exercise for practicing our pyramid and square breathing, along with breath holds (as detailed previously).

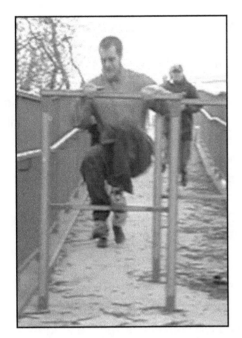

You can also incorporate obstacles into your run so you will be dodging and climbing as well. When outdoors we often get people to run through woods or forest (wear eye protection for safety). We find that it helps with awareness and also softens up the body as people have to twist, turn and change height while moving.

There is a lot to be said for running and walking outdoors in all weather conditions rather than being on a treadmill in a sterile environment. Get the wind and rain on your face!

FOOTWORK DRILLS

Aside from regular walking and running there are some specific footwork drills we can practice too. The most simple is to walk down a crowded street and not bump into anyone! But here are some more ideas.

DIRECTION CHANGE

Change direction after a certain amount of steps. It could be five steps or it could be one step. Change direction smoothly and without twisting at the knee. Keep good form. This will help develop smooth footwork

PATTERNS

Try stepping in a fixed pattern, such as a figure eight, a circle or a triangle. Once again keep good posture and smooth movement. Experiment with using these patterns against obstacles or an attacker. Another Pattern drill is to walk out letters or numbers. The basic version works like this.

Think of the numbers 1 to 9 and walk out the pattern of each of them. So for the figure 1 you would take five or so steps in straight line, figure 2 is a curve and a straight line and so on.

Now remain still and draw the figures 1 to 9 in the air with each hand in turn, then both hands at the same time. Finally, walk the figures and "air draw" them at the same time. This is basic coordination.

Now repeat the same drill but with letters instead of numbers. You can go A-Z or you can spell

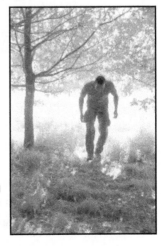

your name or similar. Once again, repeat with feet, hands, then both together.

Now comes the challenge. Draw numbers with the feet and letters with hands and vice-versa, simultaneously! This is a very good drill for developing cross-body coordination, amongst other things.

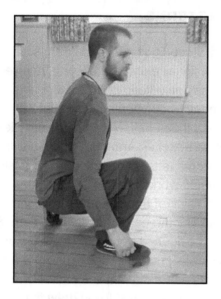

LEVEL CHANGE

Change height while walking - from upright, into a half squat, into a full squat and back up again.

Before doing this exercise be sure you can work comfortably at each level. Once again work from the hips in order not to put strain on the knees. At first it is best to pause before changing level.

So go into a full squat and try walking forwards, backwards and sideways. Keep your hips relaxed, check your foot / knee alignment and keep the back upright. Burst breathe if necessary. Then try a half squat and

work from that position. Once you are comfortable at each level, flow from one to the other whilst on the move. Make sure you are moving in a straight line when you transition, be wary of twisting, moving and changing level at this point.

It is also possible to practice "bouncing" from a full squat position, but only if you have good knees. You can work on the spot, or bounce back and forth. All the same concerns apply as for the level change.

WAVE MOVEMENT

You will sometimes see the term *wave movement* to describe types of exercise or movement pattern within Systema. The basic idea is that we allow movement to develop in one part of the body, then transfer it through to another part. In other words the body must be fluid enough to allow a force to travel through it, in any direction. This is useful for absorbing force and also for generating power for some types of striking work. Here is a simple way to begin with wave movement.

Stand in normal posture and inhale. As you exhale, push up with your right foot, raising the heel. Allow that movement to travel up the leg to the hip, which also lifts and rotates, so tilting the pelvis.

This in turn should lift the torso and chest. Then allow this movement to roll up and out of the shoulder, which lifts the arm and continues out into the hand.

In other words, there is a continuous wave of movement from the toes to the fingers. There should be no tension and no desire to put "power" into the movement, just let it happen.

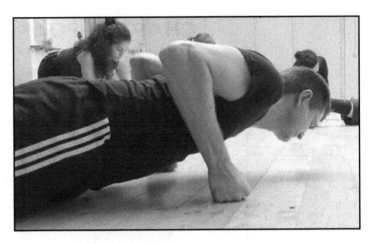

This is a basic wave movement and can be practiced with any start and end point - so one hand, across the body to the other and so on. Later on we will detail another version of this exercise which adds in breathing and tension. But for now, see if you can start a movement in one place and let it flow through you.

At first you can practice this movement in random directions. After you have the feel, try directing your movement into figure eight patterns, this will help when you move into weapons work and some types of striking. Practice slowly at first, but as you become more relaxed, begin to speed your movements up. Remember to adjust your breathing to suit

Another good way to work this, is by being pushed and going with the force. In the absence of a partner you can try bumping into and working around suitable objects. If you are feeling really brave and it is safe to do so, you could even blindfold yourself and move around your house, go slow and flow around any obstacles.

ISOLATED MOVEMENT

This is where we use the articulation of a single joint to initiate a movement. Think back to the Joint Rotation exercises we did earlier.

For simple isolated movement, stand in normal position and keep everything still. Now rotate one shoulder, so pushing out the hand.

Next try this against a wall. Place a fist on the wall and lean your weight into it. You could push yourself away by tensing the muscles of the arm, instead, roll the shoulder and see how you can move your body away. The only tension should be a little in the wrist to maintain the structure.

The same principle can be applied to push ups. Get in normal push up position and lower yourself to the floor, so the body is resting on the ground. From here, try and lift yourself without engaging the shoulder muscles. Rotate and move your shoulders in such a way that you rise with minimal muscular tension. This is a very important exercise for learning to develop powerful strikes.

CHAPTER FOUR
STRETCHING

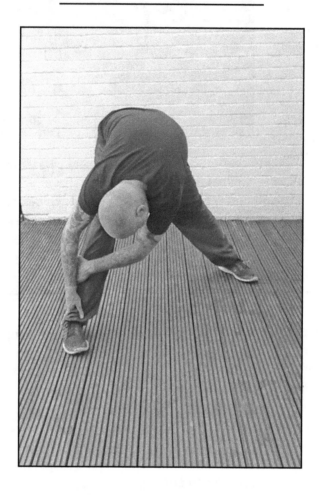

STRETCHING

Systema stretching is about releasing tension in the muscles rather than trying to "stretch tendons". It is based around overcoming the "stretch reflex".

When the muscle is taken to a point where it "feels" it is in danger it tenses in order to prevent further movement and so protect itself. When we reach that stage in the movement we should pause, inhale and tense the particular muscle as much as possible. Hold for at least 30 seconds, then sharply exhale and relax. Immediately resume the stretch and you should find you get more movement from the muscle.

Stretch slowly and with care, listen to your body. Never stretch while under tension and never "bounce", your movement should always be smooth. At the end of the stretch take your time before moving out of the exercise.

Remember, we exhale on the stretch, inhale on the return. For brevity we describe one side only, but all movements should be done on both sides

There are a huge amount of ways to stretch, we don't have the space here to cover all of them. So we have selected some basic stretches that will give you a good start. We begin with static leg stretches that you can either repeat on an inhale /exhale for a few times on each movement, or get into each position and hold, using the tense/relax breathing method described above

LEG STRETCHES

Lay on your back, legs out. Inhale and draw your heels in towards your butt. Exhale and "throw" the legs back out, they should be totally relaxed.

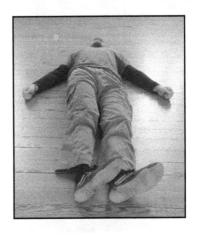

Inhale, then on the exhale pull your toes back towards your head.
Repeat a few times, then on the exhale move your feet to the left, then the right.

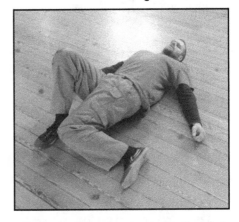

Raise both knees, keep the feet flat. On the exhale take the left knee down towards the right ankle.

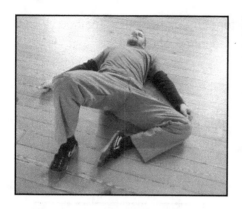

From the same position - on the exhale take the left knee outwards towards the floor.

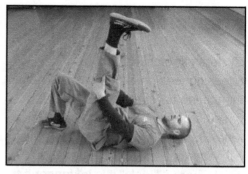

Place both hands behind the knee. Keep the leg straight and pull the knee up towards the head.

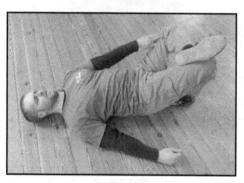

Raise both knees, feet flat on the floor. Place the left ankle onto the right knee. On the exhale, push the right knee away with the right hand

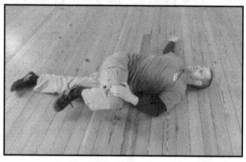

Raise the right knee. Grab it with the left hand and on the exhale pull it to the left.

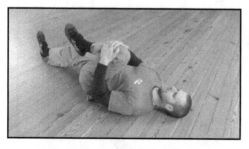

Raise the left knee. Place both hands over it and on the exhale pull the knee towards the chest.

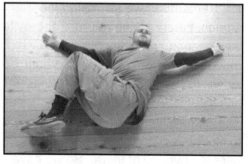

Put the arms out to the side. Bring the knees up towards the chest. On the exhale twist the legs to the left and right.

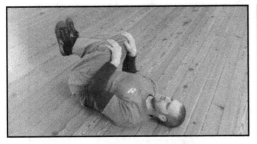

Raise the knees and place
the hands over them. Slowly rotate
the legs, in both directions and with
small and large circles.

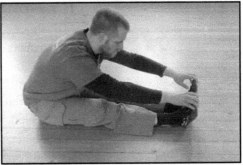

Sit with legs out in front. Lean forward
and grab the toes. Exhale and lean
forward. You may pull the toes back too.
Keep the back straight.

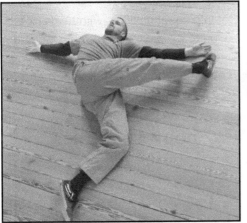

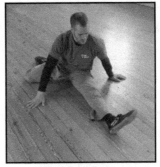

Sit in hurdle
position.
Exhale and
hold. If
comfortable
with this, on
the exhale
lean forward
and grab the
toe

Stretch arms out to the sides. Take the
right foot to the left hand on the exhale.
If possible, grab the toes and hold
the position while burst breathing.
If not simply inhale and return to start.

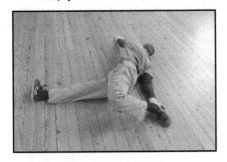

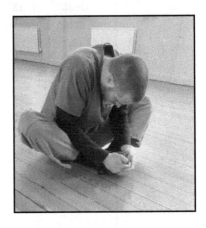

Repeat but laying on your front.
Take your time and
do it in stages if need be.

Place the soles of the feet together.
Grab the toes. On the exhale
bring the head forward and use
the elbows to push the
thighs out and down.

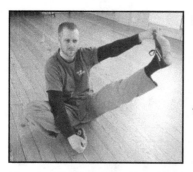

From the above position, grab the left toes with the left hand, exhale and extend the leg to the side.

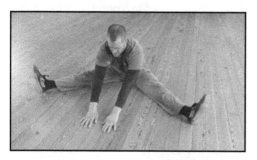

Take the feet out wide to the side. On the exhale, let the hands slide along the floor and bend forward.

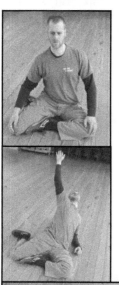

Get into the "knee walk" position described last chapter. From this posture keep the legs still and, on the exhale, bend forward, sideways and back into as many positions as you can.

Hold each with burst breathing, or return

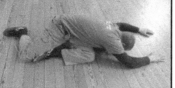

to the original posture on the inhale.

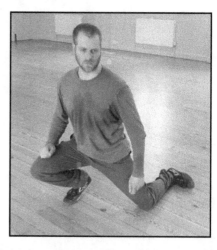

Get into squat position, with heels raised. On the exhale rotate your hip forward until your knee is on the floor. Try and keep the whole shin flat and note the position of the rear ankle.

BODY STRETCHES

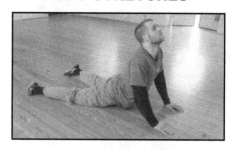

Lay on your front legs out. Inhale and relax. Exhale and raise your upper body, arching your back and lifting the head, looking up.

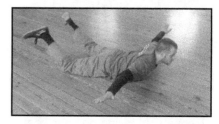

From the same start position, take your arms out to the side. On the exhale, lift the chest, arms and legs, in "parachute" style.

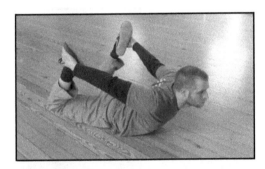

Try the same exercise again, this time grab your ankles as you lift/exhale.

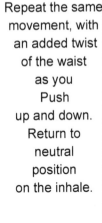

Repeat the same movement, with an added twist of the waist as you Push up and down. Return to neutral position on the inhale.

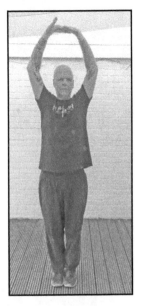

With palms facing up, push the hands up towards the ceiling as high as you can, on an exhale. You may also raise the heels at the same time.

Place the hand behind the neck and reach over to grab the elbow with the opposite hand. On the exhale, pull the elbow across.

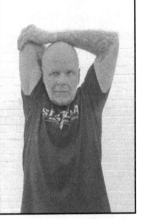

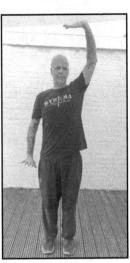

Repeat, but this time one hand pushes up as the other pushes down, Note the position of the fingers, low hand forward, upper hand to the side.

Reach across the body, arm straight. Place the opposite forearm outside the elbow. Exhale, pull the elbow in and allow the shoulders and back to relax and open.

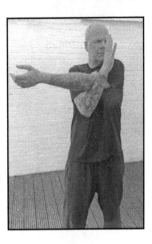

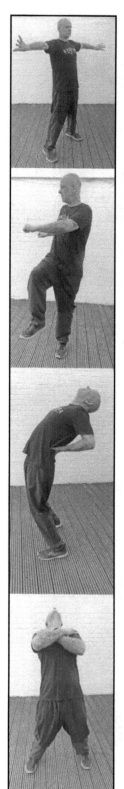

Take the arms out to the sides, palms up. On the exhale, twist the arms so the palms rotate 180 degrees. Try with arms forward and back.

Hold the arms out, bent at 90 degrees, each hand makes a fist. On the exhale twist to the side and lift the foot. Try taking the right hand to the left knee and vice versa.

Place the palms in the small of the back and inhale. Exhale and slowly bend back. Do not go too far at first and check before attempting if you have a back problem.

Cross the hands over the chest and inhale. On the exhale bend back, as above.

Also try bending to the side and forwards.

Exhale, bend the body to the side and grab the ankle with one or both hands. Pull the chin towards the knee. Try and keep the back straight.

Place the back of the wrist against the side. Grab the elbow with the opposite hand. Inhale.

On the exhale, pull the elbow gently across. Hold for a few seconds, then return to the start point.

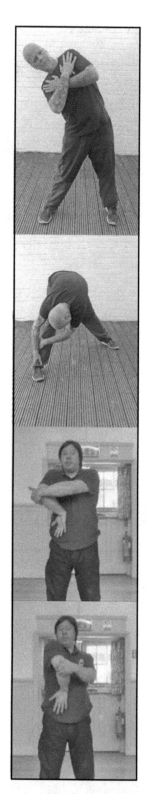

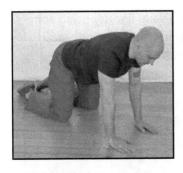

Place hands and knees on the floor, under the shoulders and hips. Keep the back level, do not let it sag or arch.

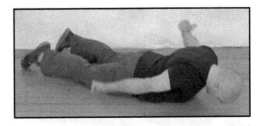

Sweep your hands up and back as you exhale.

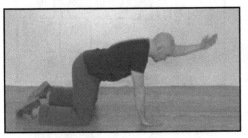

Without shifting the weight, extend one arm out and forward. Bring it back and repeat with the other arm.
Now carry out the same movement with each leg in turn.

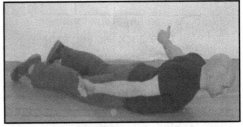

Continue the inhale as you rotate the thumbs upward and allow the chest to lift off the ground.
Do not force the move and keep the head pointing forward, do not tilt the neck. Exhale and return to the start position.

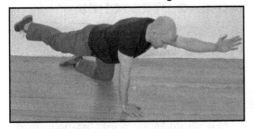

Extend the opposite arm and leg at the same time. Don't forget to exhale on the movement.

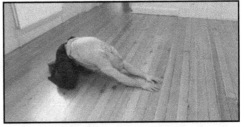

Kneel on the floor and let your hips relax. As you exhale, take your hands forward to the floor and slide them out as far as they will go.
Let the lower back and shoulders relax and open.
Hold with burst breathing then return to the start point.

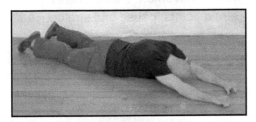

Lie on your front with arms extended forward. Keep the head down. Inhale.

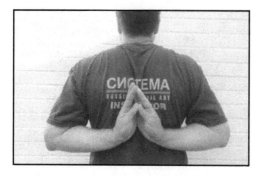

Place the fingertips together behind the back. As you exhale push the palms together and lift the hands as far as you can up the back.
If you can, get the hands between the shoulder blades. Hold and burst breath, while pulling back your elbows and shoulders.

Bridging is a more challenging exercise and we recommend taking it in stages.
Start by laying on the floor, arms at sides. Bring the knees in, feet flat on the ground and, on the exhale, raise the pelvis up. Keep your shoulders on the floor.

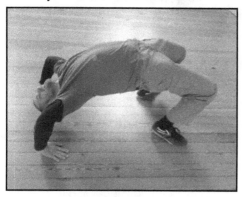

If this is comfortable, try the full bridge. Start as above, but place the palms on the floor, fingers pointing towards your feet. Exhale and push up.

If you struggle at first, try using some support under the body, or get a partner to assist.

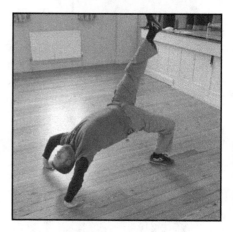

Once you can do the above well, try adding in variations, such as raising the leg, moving around and so on. But always exercise care!

MOVING STRETCHES

So far we have looked at static stretches. But it is also possible to combine your stretching into a movement routine. Remember how we spoke about Movement Chains in the section on Ground Movement?
What you do is run through your ground movement chains and at certain points, pause and stretch. This

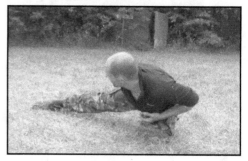

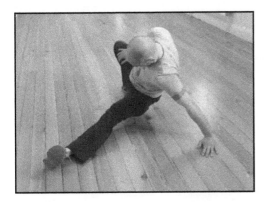

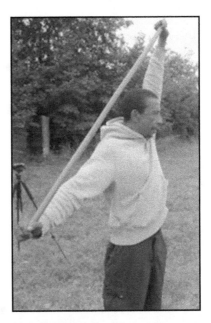

also means you learn to use the static stretch positions as start and end points for ground movement, or sometimes as a transition.

You can also experiment with using the hand or foot to initiate the

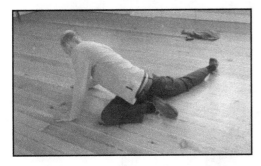

movement. In other words, the hand or foot leads and the rest of the body follows.

Don't be afraid to experiment and try to incorporate stretches from difficult or odd positions. Once again, this will break you out of the "norm" of stretching and help make all of your work dynamic and fluid.

EQUIPMENT

One last thing to mention is the use of equipment for stretching. There are numerous "stretching machines" on the market. Personally, I have never used one, but if you find they work for you, then go for it. What I have found useful, however are some of the everyday objects you find around you. For leg stretches, use a chair or table to rest your ankle on, then practice touching the toes, etc.

The ever-reliable stick is another useful tools for stretching. Use it for the upper body / shoulders, or use it for a leg stretch by sitting and placing the stick between the ankles in order to help push them apart.

Other specialist equipment worth checking out includes yoga wheels, to help with back arches, or similar. Whatever equipment you decide to use, however, always remember the aim of stretching is to decrease tension and increase freedom of movement, not to become a circus act! Extreme methods may produce spectacular results, but often at the expense of long term health.

CHAPTER FIVE
EQUIPMENT

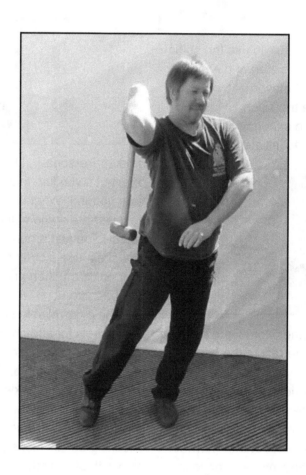

EQUIPMENT

Mention equipment and solo training and most people will naturally think of the gym. However there are many other things we can use in order to develop strength, sensitivity and other attributes. We should also consider how working with equipment such as fixed weights will only develop us in one plane of movement. In order to be adaptable we should be strong in all ranges of motion.

When using equipment, especially heavy items, always put safety first. Be aware of your surroundings and never train any heavy item to failure. Start with comfortable repetitions and increase slowly. The use of good posture and breathing should go without saying – always breathe when working tension under load!

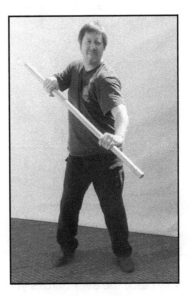

Move the stick around in circular or figure eight patterns. Use a double or single hand grip, switching from left to right and vice versa. Keep movements relaxed and smooth.

THE STICK

The stick is the single most useful piece of kit for Systema solo training (and for many partner drills too!). The stick should be around 4 foot long and quite thick. I find a cut down curtain pole or similar works well. A broomstick is ok for some exercises, but is not strong enough for load bearing.

Make sure you have enough space to work with the stick! Always check your surroundings and be aware of anyone or anything around you.

The first thing to do with your stick, is simply to get used to the feel of it.

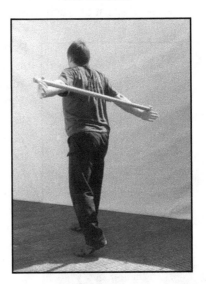

Now raise the stick above your head and see if you can take it over your head and down behind you. Repeat this movement back and forth a few times.

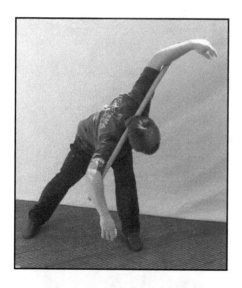

Keep the stick parallel to the floor, release and grip it, each time moving your hand along the stick. Exhale as you grip and keep the fist strong. If necessary, enlist the aid of a small cat.

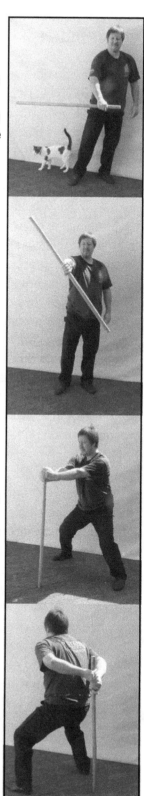

Now place the stick across your shoulders and hang your elbows over it. Twist the body to the left and the right and also make circles / figure eights.
Following this, lean forward and take your hand towards the opposite knee. Repeat on each side.

Hold the stick in the centre and twist the wrist from left to right. You can do this quite quickly

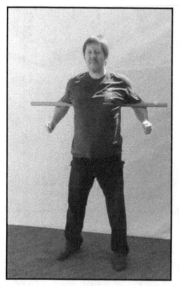

Perform the same moves with the stick held behind the back and across the chest. You can also hold in this position and tense the arms

Place the stick upright, bend the knees. Tense the arms and push the stick down into the ground as hard as you can. Burst breathe and keep the body relaxed.

as though trying to break the stick across the body (use burst breathing)

Place the stick behind you, in the same way and repeat.

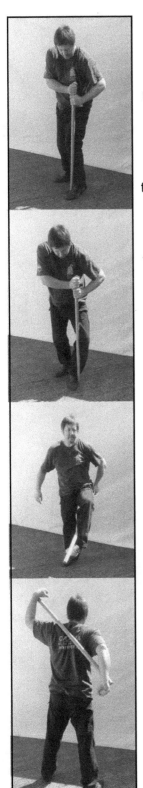

Place the stick inside the foot and outside the knee.
Using tension in the leg, push against the stick as though you are trying to break it. Burst breathe.

Repeat with the stick outside of the foot and inside the knee.

Repeat once more with the stick under the thigh and over the top of the foot.

Place the stick across the back. Push the raised arm forward, as though trying to break the stick. Let the lower arm relax and move back slightly. Following this, switch the push to the lower hand and allow the upper hand to relax.

Hold the stick in front at waist height. Grip it tightly and, with tension in the forearms, push inwards along the stick.

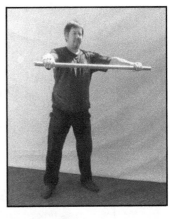

Maintain the tension and slowly lift the stick above the head, while burst breathing. Once you are above the head, relax. Then tense the arms, push once more and lower to start position.

Repeat, this time pulling on the ends of the stick. Following this, repeat both movements with the stick held behind you.

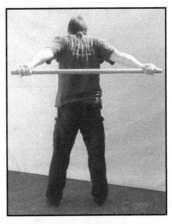

Rest the end of the stick against a wall. Keep the body straight and "climb" up and down the stick,

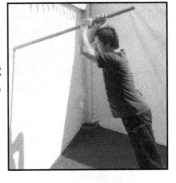

with burst breathing. Allow the heels to lift so all your weight is on the stick.

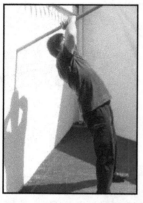

Do not go too far down at first and be sure you can keep the stick in place.

Repeat with the stick behind you. Once again, do not go too far down the stick at first and be sure to keep the body straight.

Hold the stick out in front of you at chest height. Relax and rotate the shoulders, then the chest, while keeping the hands in place.

Swing the stick across to one side, reversing the grip on the upper hand as you do so.

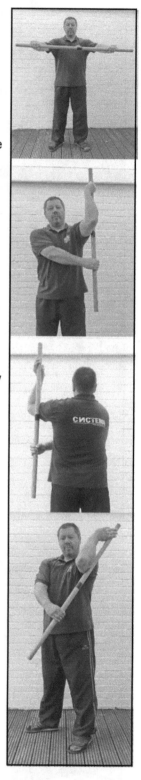

Reverse view

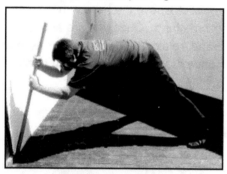

You can then try the same exercise but with the stick supported in a corner

From here pull the lower hand forward and allow the shoulder to relax . This is a good exercise for the rotator cuff. You can also experiment with different hand and stick positions.

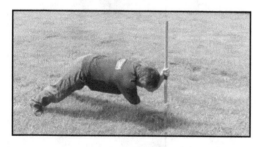

Another variation is to place the stick upright on the ground and then climb up and down it. You can do this with the stick to the front and also with it behind you, from a sitting position.
With each of these exercises, be sure that you use a stick capable of bearing your weight.

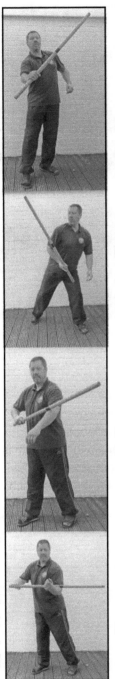

Hold the stick in one hand and begin to move it around. At first keep to a simple pattern, such as an up/down or left right movement.

You can then begin to work things like a large X shape, or a Figure Eight pattern. Keep the stick moving smoothly at all times, there should be no break in movement.

Allow the body to relax and get a feel for using the momentum of the stick and a roll of the shoulders and hips to power the movement. Don't put any tension into the "strikes".

Allow the stick to contact the body and when it does, absorb then "push out" to keep the stick moving.

So if the stick contacts the arm, then fold the elbow in to absorb, then flick out to bounce the stick away. The same movement applies to shoulders, legs, or any other part of the body.

Work on the spot at first, then begin moving around - if you have the space!

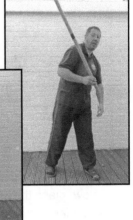

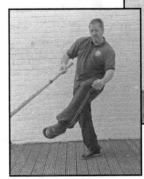

We can also use the stick on the ground At first, place the stick on the floor and being to roll and move around and over it.

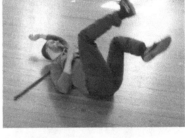

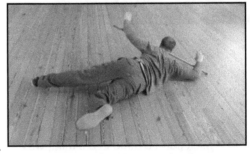

Now perform your regular ground movements but while holding the stick in various ways. Start by holding the stick in your hands, both close to the body and then with outstretched arms.
Explore how you can use the stick to assist your movement, by pushing with one end of it against the floor and so on.

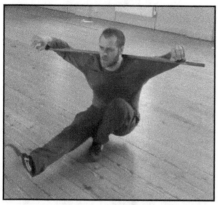

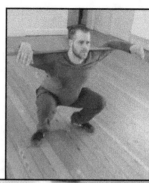

leg raise and squats. Experiment with different hand and stick positions.

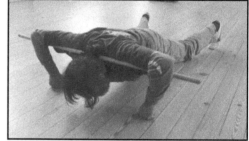

Now place the stick across your shoulders. Try moving on the floor in this position.
Then practice going from standing to the floor and up again, working to the front and to the back.

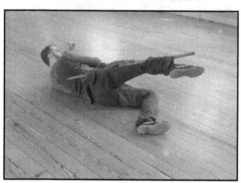

THE CHAIN

Where the stick gives us something solid to work with, the chain is flexible and so present new challenges!
The best type of chain to work with is from your local hardware store. It should be quite heavy, with links about an inch or so long and the whole chain should be around three or four feet in length.

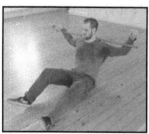

For another challenge, try placing the stick down the leg of your pants! Now try ground movement, getting up, falling, rolling etc

The stick can be used in a similar way with the Core Exercises. Once again, place the stick across the shoulders and perform your push ups, sit ups,

The first thing to do is to get used to the feel of the chain. Hold one end of the chain and feel the weight of it, move around a little and swing the chain slowly.

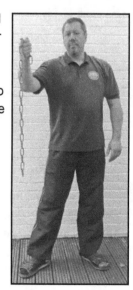

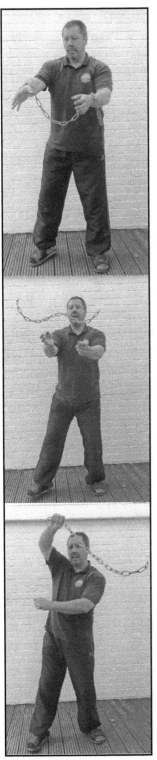

Now let the chain hang over your wrists and move your arms around a little. Raise and lower the hands, feeling how the chain slides up and down the arms.

Place the chain across the wrists once more, now throw the chain up and catch it across the arms.

Following this hold the end of the chain in one hand and begin making slow movements. Of course, check your surroundings first!

Make circles, figure eights or any kind of movement and see how the chain responds. Next, swing the chain from one side to another and "catch it" on the inside of your opposite arm. As the chain hits the arm, bring the elbow in towards the body in order to absorb the force, as we did with the stick earlier, then flick it back out.

Try the same movement against the body. Swing the chain quite hard and as it hits, move the body to absorb the strike, then flick it back out again. You can also do the same against the legs.

Finally, allow the chain to slide around the body. Don't use the hands to guide, just use the movement of shoulders, etc.

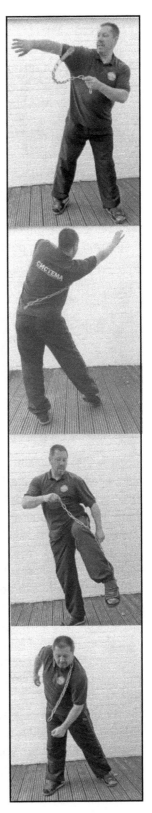

THE HAMMER

When strength training comes up, the use of weights is always an issue. We've already mentioned fixed weights in the gym and how they are primarily used to develop "local" muscle, sometimes purely for aesthetic purposes.

So let us consider free weights. After all, we can take those gym weights and use them "freestyle". That is one option. Another free weight option that has become increasing popular are kettlebells (KBs). In fact KBs are now so

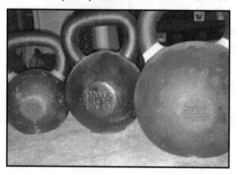

popular that a Russian tradition has in some cases become acquired by other martial art styles! I'm all for taking ideas from wherever you can, but please give credit where it is due. The same applies for many Systema movements and exercises, but I digress!

Personally I have never used KBs, so have not included them here, besides which there are a huge amount of resources available for good KB training. Be sure to find an original source though and not one of the "we do it because it's trendy" schools!

Opinion does vary about the use of weights. The old stereotype is that too much weights makes you big and slow. This may be the case for some, but I have known people who had both bulk

and speed and flexibility. However, they took a very balanced approach to training and always worked to offset the tension created by "pure" weight training.

Personally, for weight training I have always favoured the use of weapons, such as sword and staff, and the sledgehammer. To my mind there is a very clear connection between sword and sledgehammer work and, indeed, between the hammer and certain methods of punching.

So for me, the sledgehammer is purely functional weight training, which develops not only strength for a movement, but also the basic patterns of movement for application. That application is beyond our remit here, but you can test this out for yourself simply by working the sledgehammer movements empty hand against focus pads.

Two words of warning before we start. The first is about tension - be sure to always breath when carrying out the movements and keep the body as relaxed as possible. Do not do these exercises to failure! And of course, balance them out with all your other training.

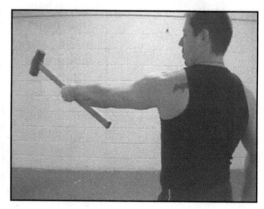

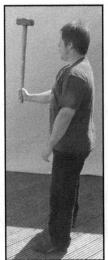

The second point is safety. Be sure you have enough room and start every new movement with care. I suggest at first, all you do is pick up the hammer near the head and carry it around, get a feel for the weight and the leverage - because it is the leverage that can catch you out! Start every exercise near the head and move down the handle as you improve.

Weight wise, all you need is a standard 7lb hammer from your local hardware store. Don't be macho and get anything heavier, I've had guys turn up with long handled 14lb hammers before and they couldn't even lift them - waste of time!

In fact, I would advise that you start with a regular small hammer or even a stick. The main thing initially is to get the mechanics correct and add the weight in after.

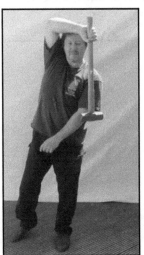

For our first exercise, hold the hammer parallel to the body and circle it around yourself. Involve the whole body in the movement, so the feet, hips and shoulders all articulate. Keep your movement slow and relaxed. Don't forget to breath.

After a few repetitions, stop and circle back the other way, following the same procedure.

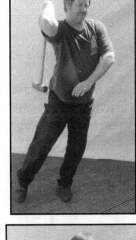

Finish by placing the hammer back on the floor. You can work this circular movement with a single grip, or with both hands holding the hammer.

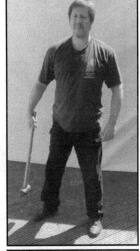

For our next exercise, bring the hammer up from the floor to a 90 degree angle, in one smooth movement and hold it in place for a couple of seconds. At first it is best to grip the handle closer up to the head.

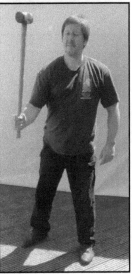

Use a wave motion as we described in the earlier chapter. So the movement is initiated in the feet and travels through the hip, body and shoulder out along the arm. You can step forward as you lift.

Later, you can use the isolated movement of the hip in order to lift the hammer. Remember to exhale on the lift!

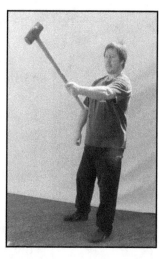

shoulder helping to lift, or as an isolated movement, purely from the shoulder. Be sure to start well up the handle, at first. Once again, exhale on the lift, inhale on the return.

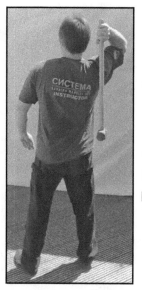

The second exercise is, from the last upright position, take the hammer back over your shoulder, to hang down. Then return back to the 90 degree position and hold. You can practice these moves separately, or link them together - so, lift from the floor to 90 degrees, take back over the shoulder, return to 90 degrees, then back to rest on the floor

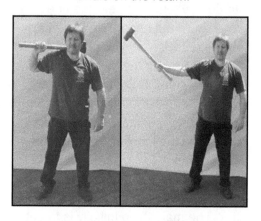

The next exercise is similar, but we move the hammer out to the side, rather than forward.

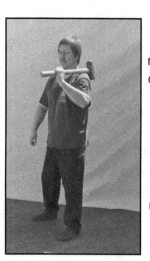

Our next exercise is to rest the hammer on the shoulder, then move it out to a 45 degree angle and hold. Again we can use a wave movement, with rotation of the

Next, hold the head of the hammer in line with the centre of the chest. Inhale and expand the chest, lifting the hammer out to the side. Exhale and let the chest sink

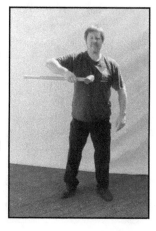

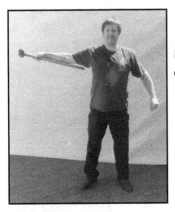

and the shoulder blades open out, bringing the hammer back to the start point. Keep the handle tight along the forearm.

Hold the hammer out in front of you with hand at chest height. Tilt the fist so the head of the hammer moves back and forward. On the forward tilt, exhale and open the

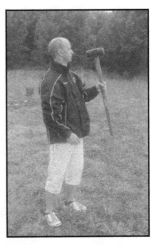

shoulder blades out. Inhale and squeeze them together on the back tilt.
Try and power the movement from the back as much as you can.
You can try the same movement, but move the handle and try and keep the hammer head in the same place.

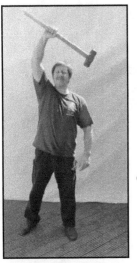

For the next exercise, lift the hammer and circle it. You can either circle it with the head down, keeping the hammer close to the body, or you can try and keep the handle above the head.

These are some of the basic movements that you can work with the hammer. Once you have a good feel for them and are confident with the weight and leverage, begin blending the movements together, in much the same way as we did with the ground movement exercises earlier.

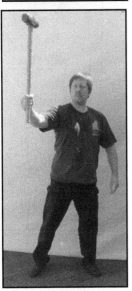

Whichever way you try, from that movement bring the hammer out upright in front of you, with your hand at shoulder height, on an exhale.

So you may flow from lifting the hammer to the floor, bring it up over the head, out to the front, then to the shoulder lift and so on. You should also explore different movement patterns, as we do with the stick - circles, Figure Eights and so on.

Think of the hammer as a weapon and of the ways you could use it to strike, block and deflect and you will get plenty of ideas for freestyle movements.

THE BALL

For this book we will show you some simple exercises with a tennis ball and football. For an excellent series of drills with a medicine ball, we recommend you get Martin Wheeler's download on this subject, available via his website.

A ball can also be a useful tool for health / massage work and we will cover that use later on. For now, let us start with some tactile sensitivity work.

Try this exercise with a football, a children's play ball and also a tennis ball.

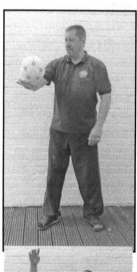

Place the ball on the back of the hand / forearm and keep it in place. Move the feet and body around as you need to in order the maintain contact and not let the ball drop.

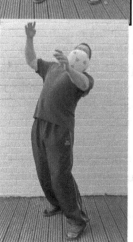

Then begin to allow the ball to roll around the body, again do not let it drop. For added challenge, walk around, change level and so on.

Now work against a wall. Trap the ball between the wall and your arm and allow the ball to move. Follow the movement and do not let the ball drop. Once you have this idea, repeat, but contact the ball with different parts of the body, the shoulder, back, etc.

From there, try transferring the contact point from one part of the body to another, without letting the ball drop. You should try and keep the touch light with these exercises and allow your body to follow the movement of the ball. You can also work the same method on the ground.

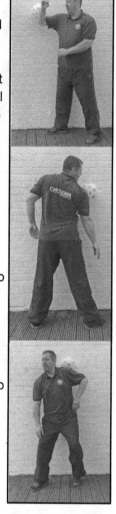

Now take the football again and hold it in both hands. Stay on the spot and rotate the ball around in the hands, keeping contact with it at all times. Start walking while doing the same movements. After a while, start level changing, go into squat, all the way to the floor and up again while rotating the ball in the hands. Don't grab the ball and keep your touch as light as possible. Finally go to the floor and move around in the same way.

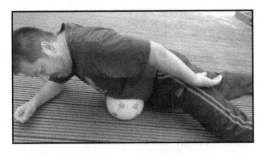

Place any size ball on the floor and put your body weight onto it. Move around while keeping contact with the ball. Let it guide your movement and keep fluid and relaxed. Work on your front, back and each side in turn

WEAPONS

Weapons have an obvious practical application, for offence and defence. However, they are also very useful for solo training. You may use this training in order to prepare for the weapon's use, or simply in order to develop attributes.

When working with weapons, particularly blades, we should be even more aware of safety issues. Never start training with a sharp weapon. Be aware of your surroundings. Do not jump into doing movements that may cause harm. Take it steady and slow.

We have already covered some ideas of training with the stick and, to some extent, you can replicate many of the sword, knife and even gun movements with different lengths of stick. Again, this is a good, safe starting point to get you into the movement.

So let us begin by looking at bladed weapons.

THE KNIFE

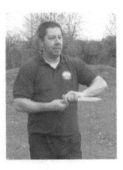

If you want to start training with a metal blade straight away, we recommend using a simple butter knife with a rounded end.

This will give you the feel of metal but should be fairly blunt. Start simply by handling the knife, trying different grips and moving it from hand to hand.

Once you have a feel for the weapon, go through the handling again, this time on the move. Walk around, change level, work on the ground.

Hold the knife close to the body.

Slide your other hand between the blade and your body and transfer the knife to the other hand.

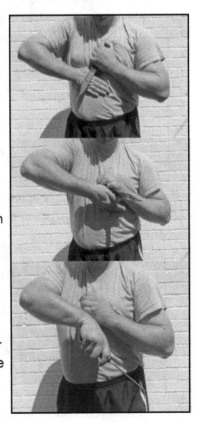

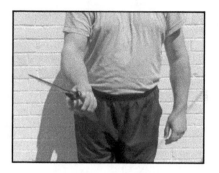

Hold the knife point up in front of you.

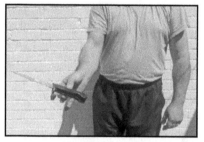

Loosen your grip and hold the knife
with thumb and middle finger.

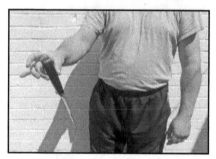

Move your hand sharply up and across,
allowing the knife to rotate to point down.

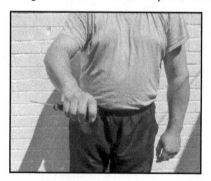

Close your fingers around
the handle again

Now try the same movement again. From the reverse grip, once again swing the knife out between thumb and middle finger.

Flick the hand to rotate the knife and bring it back into the forward grip.

You should practice this move back and forward until it is smooth.

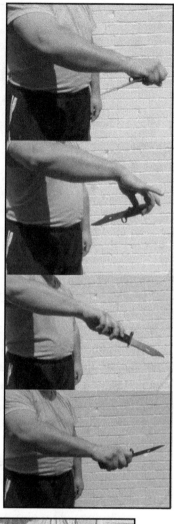

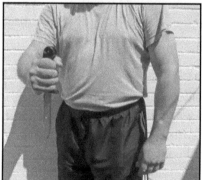

Now hold the knife out in front of
you, blade down. Bring the back
of your free hand up to
contact the blade.

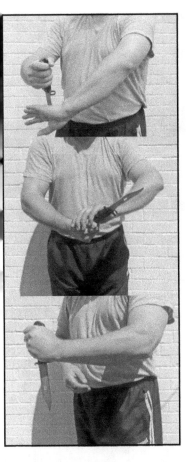

Push the hand back, rotating the blade towards you and up.

This should bring the handle up into the free hand.

Repeat the process, bring the knife back to the original hand.

Once again, practice this move repeatedly until it is smooth and fluid.

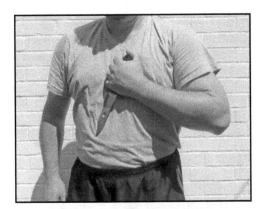

Place the blade flat against the body. Now move the knife around the body, keeping the blade flat.

See how you can move the blade with body movement, much the same as we did with the chain. Try working without grabbing the knife too much, keep the body as loose as possible.

Also practice holding the knife in different parts of the body, such as the crook of the elbow, under the arm and so on.

This is not only a good drill to work body movement, it also gets you used to the feel of the blade, from a physical and psychological perspective

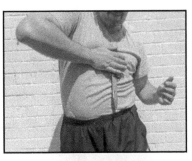

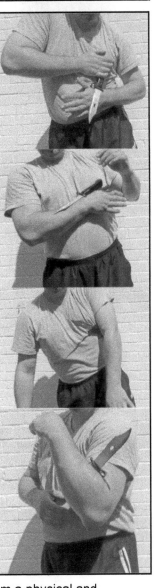

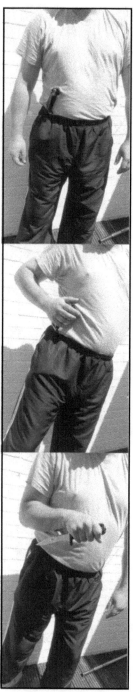

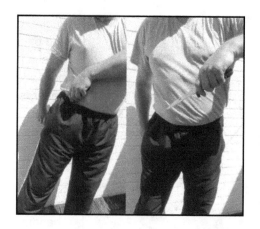

Place the knife in the belt. Practice drawing the knife from a static, standing position.

One way to do this is to use a rotation of the hip in order to draw the knife. This method makes your draw very difficult to jam.

You should also practice the same thing with a cross-body draw.

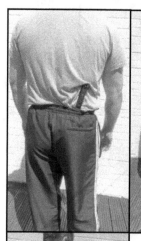

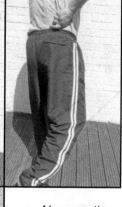

Simply bring the hip up so that the knife is moved towards the hand.

Grasp the handle, then let the hip drop down. It is this action which draws the knife, rather than a pulling of the hand.

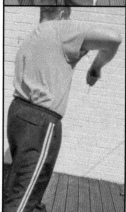

Also practice the draw with the knife at your back. See how the leg moves in order to assist the draw.

For the hip rotation, think back to the walking exercise where we practiced lifting the foot by rotating the hip - it is the same movement.

Once you can do this smoothly in a static position, add in an evasive body movement. Try and make it all one movement, rather than "evade and draw". Think back to the body wave we spoke about earlier.

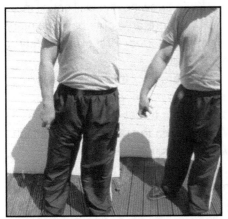

Palm the knife in one hand, keeping the blade parallel to the forearm.

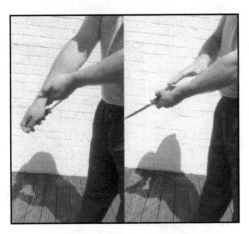

Slide the other hand along the forearm and transfer the knife into it.

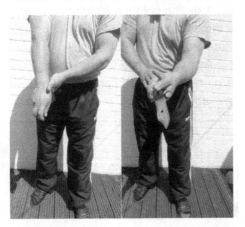

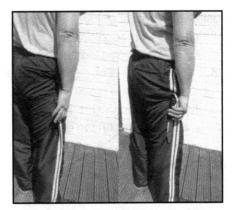

Fold the knife into your trouser leg. Let the knife drop into the hand.

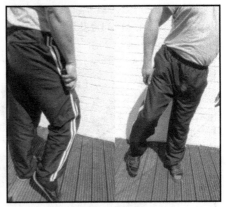

Shift the leg aside to bring the knife out and forward.

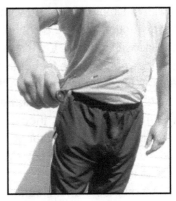

These are some methods of deploying a knife. While we do not condone use of a knife unless absolutely necessary, it is vital to understand how the knife can be deployed from hidden positions as part of our knife defence training. It is also good practice for developing knife handling attributes. Once you can do these draws smoothly, practice them on the move, while walking, while going to the floor and finally while moving on the ground.

CUTTING

If you would like to practice cutting with a knife, first find a stick or similar that can be safely cut. You can either fix it in place or have a friend hold it in a safe position. It is best for everyone to wear thick gloves at first.

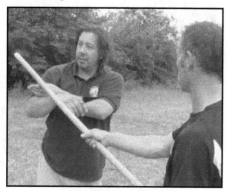

Begin with a simple up and down cutting motion, as though you are painting a straight line with a brush. Let the wrist relax. Once you have the feel of this, add a little more shoulder in and make the movement more circular, or a figure eight. Start with big circles, then work smaller. Carry out the same exercises, but with a lateral cut. Work both hands in each case.

Once comfortable and, if safe, work on cutting straight from the draw. Then work on walking in and cutting. Finally, with safety in mind, have a partner thrust the stick towards you, evade, draw and cut in on fluid move.

THROWING

Knife throwing is a skill set all in itself, but here are some basic pointers to get you started. First of all - safety once again!

Be sure your throwing area is free from pets and people. Check what is behind your target, in case you miss it! Working with the target against a high wall or similar is best.

Also be aware that your knife may rebound from the target back towards you. Anyone not throwing should stay behind you and out of the line of fire. Make sure you are wearing suitable clothing, in particular do not throw barefoot, in case of drops or rebounds.

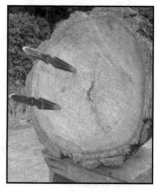

In terms of target, there are numerous commercial targets available. If you do not want to use one of these, you may find a something like an old door or tabletop can be used. It should be something that will take and hold the knife point when it is thrown correctly. Softwood is the best material.

As to what knife to use - there are a large number of "proper" throwing knives available, it is best to start with those.

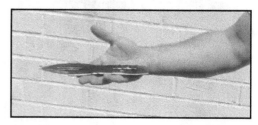

Find some who size and weight suits you. We advise having at least three or four knives as you will soon get fed up walking backwards and forward to the target! After a while you should experiment throwing any type of knife, from a kitchen knife to a "combat" knife, and everything inbetween.

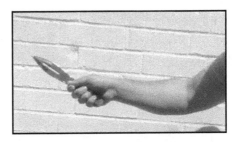

At first practice getting into a comfortable position, around six feet away far from the target. We 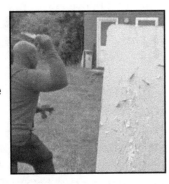 recommend that at first you do not even use a knife, but throw a tennis ball or similar, to get a feel for posture and distance.

Stand slightly side on to the target, with your throwing hand to the rear. Let's assume the ball is in your right hand. Step out a little with your left foot, bring the right hand up to your ear.

Pivot the waist and throw the ball overhand at the target. You should be able to hit the target easily, if not check your posture and make sure you are not twisting the waist to much, or releasing the ball at the wrong time. Once you can do this, you can start working with the knife.

Hold the knife with a relaxed grip, point upwards. As you rotate the waist just let the arm travel forward to throw the blade, do not flick the wrist. At this distance you want the knife to make one complete rotation before sticking into the

target. You may have to work with adjusting your range slightly, or the amount of strength your are putting into the throw. There shouldn't be too much power in the throw, let the movement and the rotation do the job. If you put too much tension and speed in at first, you will find it difficult to get impact with the point. Remember smooth is fast!

Once you can get a consistent rate of hits you can start adjusting distance. As you move further back you might find you need to put a bit more "spin" into the throw and get two or three rotations.

This may take some time and there is no substitute for practice! However after a while you will find you can hit the target point on with a good percentage of your throws. Now you can try working with different types of knife. You will note that every blade has a different balance, weight and so on that

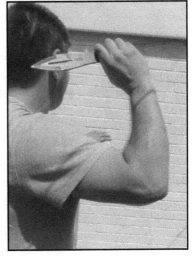

you will need to make adjustments for. But it doesn't have to be knives. You can try throwing nails, spikes, throwing stars, even axes and shovels.

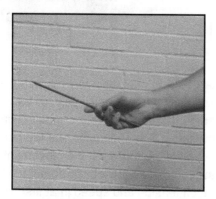

Once you have static throwing down, add in some movement. Take a few steps back, then throw on the walk or run in. Take a dive, then throw as you come up out of the roll .

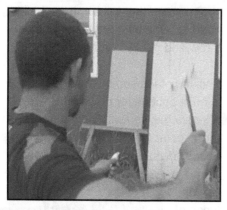

Start with your back to the target, turn and throw in one move. If you have the space and facilities you can set up a run with targets at different heights and positions through it.

This is a brief introduction to the art of knife throwing. For more information and ideas, check out the numerous tutorials, available or, even better, get in some time with an experienced thrower!

THE SWORD

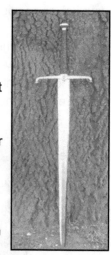

Sword methods vary in line with the martial and cultural traditions they have been developed in, but there are some underlying principles that hold true whatever the background or style.

Our aim here is not to give you an in-depth training regime for a specific style of sword play, but instead to explore some basic, universal movements that will help you become familiar with handling the weapon and develop some good attributes. As with the knife, we recommend working with a stick first, then a blunt training weapon and, finally an edged blade if you wish to. All the usual safety precautions apply of course.

The first question is - what type of sword? We can broadly divide swords into slashing or stabbing. So a rapier is designed to stab, while a cutlass is generally a slashing weapon. Of course, some swords can do both!
As we are studying a Russian martial art is seems appropriate to use a Cossack sabre, or *shaskka*. However many of the same moves are also seen with the Chinese *Dao*, the English sabre and so on.

Once again, further research and training is available from a variety of sources if you wish to explore a particular sword tradition in greater detail.

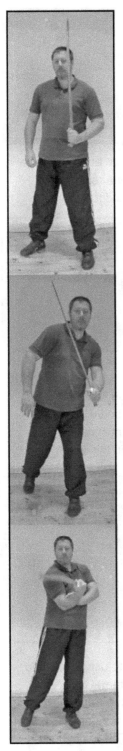

Our process starts once again with basic handling. Hold the sword in a comfortable grip and get used to its weight and balance.

Start by making simple X shaped cuts in front of you. Keep your movements large and clear. As you get comfortable, add more body movement in so that the X becomes a Figure Eight.

Remember, the power comes from the body movement, not from tension.

Once you are ok on one side, switch hands and start again.

Try the same patterns again, but make the circles much smaller.

Now, think back to the sledgehammer exercises and you will see how they relate to sword as well as empty hand movements. Try some of the hammer moves with the sword.

The only difference is that instead of holding the position, you want to be slicing through as though cutting into an object.

So, for example, circle the sword around the head, in a parrying movement, then cut forward.

Take up a neutral position. Flick the arm up and back to stab behind you. Then circle into an overhead cut.

Practice this until smooth on both sides. Then you can start varying the movements.

For example, rather than a downward slice, bring the sword round and into an upward cut.

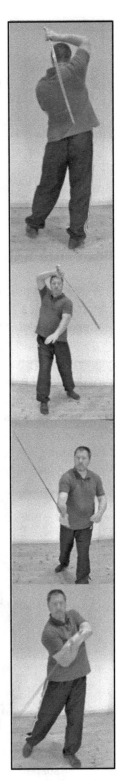

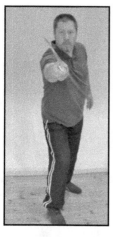

Continue this into a Figure Eight pattern, then stab forward and back.

Let the movement of the sword guide you at this stage, just guide it to where it wants to go.

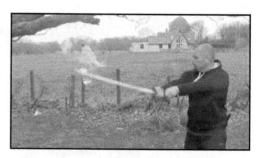

Make sure you have enough space and of course, we recommend being outdoors!

CUTTING AND STABBING

We can practice sword cutting along the same lines as the knife, with all the attendant safety factors in place. Of course, you will need a live blade for cutting work and should be confident in handling the sword prior to undertaking any cutting work.

In terms of target, you can use a stick or pole as before. One thing we have found very useful for cutting are plastic drinks bottles.

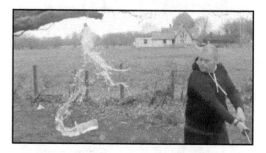

Swing and cut. If you have good form and movement you should make a clear cut of the bottle. You can practice different slashes and also stabs in this way.

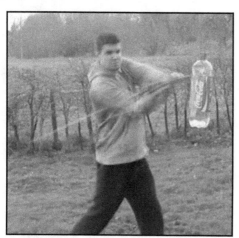

Get a large, empty bottle and fill it with water. Put the top on and suspend the bottle from a convenient place.

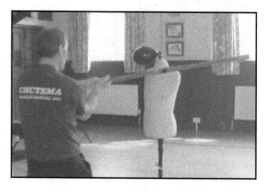

Another option is to use some kind of dummy as a target. You can practice strikes with a training sword, or use something like bamboo rods bound together. This way you can safely put power into your movements.

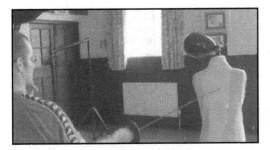

This type of dummy can also be used to practice stabs. Balloons make another good target.

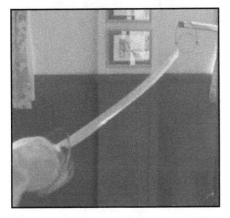

A god method to practice stabs is to make some loops out of wire and hang them from a suitable object. See if you can stab the blade through the loop without touching the wire.

FIREARMS

Firearms are obviously another area of specialised training. If you are serious about learning their use, we strongly advise seeking out a reputable shooting club or similar qualified instruction.

Outside of that, in the context of solo training with firearms, there are two aspects to consider. One is how our regular movement can be incorporated into firearms use. The second is the technical aspects of shooting.

It is entirely possible to use firearms purely as a tool for movement skills. To this end, you can easily work with a replica gun, such as the rubber one illustrated below.

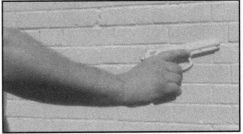

A replica will give you some feel or focus for your movement, while at the same time being wholly legal (but please check local laws) and completely safe. So let's start with some simple movement and handling with the pistol. Of course, if legal, you can practice the same with a replica rifle.

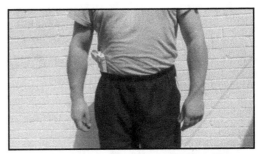

Handle the weapon and get used to the weight and feel. Place the gun in the belt and practice drawing, in much the same way as we did with the knife earlier.

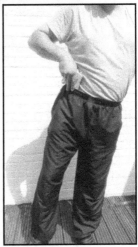

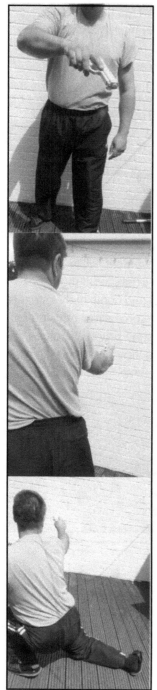

Remember to lift the hip to bring the gun to the hand. Practice this movement static and then on the move. You can then add in level changes and working on the ground.

Point the gun at a particular spot on the wall. Walk left, right, back and forward while keeping the gun trained on the spot. Allow the body to be relaxed and fluid.

Carry out the same movement while changing level. Then go to the ground and maintain the aim whilst moving on the floor.

SHOOTING

As we mentioned before, to learn how to handle and use firearms properly and safely, you must seek out qualified instruction. In the UK it is easy, and legal at time of writing, to use Airsoft guns to train, providing they meet current legislation requirements. Make sure all safety procedures are in place.

There are a huge range of Systema drills you can practice with Airsoft weapons, we recommend the materials available from Systema HQ, particularly the work of Konstantin Komarov.

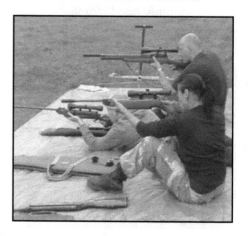

For a few quick ideas, start with basic, static target work.

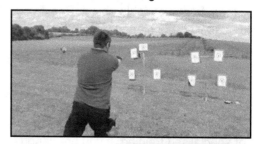

From here you can move onto rapid shooting at multiple targets. The next step is adding in level changes and shooting from different positions.

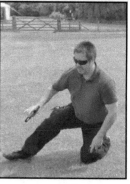

THE SHOVEL

The military shovel is a tool that has become synonymous with Spetsnaz, but is used by military forces around the world. Its design is such that it has a multitude of as a weapon.

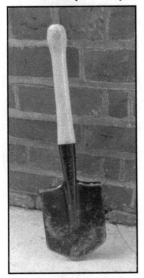

You can get military shovels from most army surplus outfits. If you want the specific Russian design a quick hunt around the Internet should turn up a supplier.

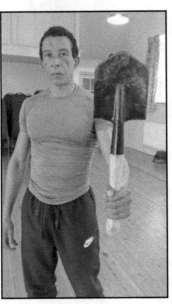

Solo training with the shovel follows the same procedures as the other weapons we have looked at. Start by simply handling the shovel and getting used to its weight and balance.

After this, start making simple X shape cutting movements, developing into Figure Eights. Work through the same progression as with the knife, stick, etc,

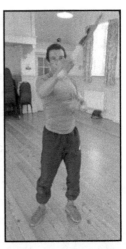

Large movements to small, static to mobile, level change and working on the ground.

You can also practice throwing the shovel. Try overarm, underarm, static and moving, as with he knife.

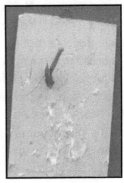

I'm sure you see by now that there is a simple template for using any weapon in solo training. This is not the same as learning how to use the weapon necessarily, but will , at the very least, develop confidence in handling, an idea of safety procedures and a level of psychological comfort in weapons work.

This procedure is applicable to any object, so be adaptable in your training. On a practical level this will help you develop the ability to use almost anything to hand as a weapon, be it flexible, fixed, bladed or missile.

In each case if you wish to take things further, seek out qualified instruction, you may even discover new hobbies such as archery, shooting and so on.

ENVIRONMENT

Our last area of Equipment use is to look at what we have around us and see if it can be used to help our training. This has two advantages. The first is that you begin to develop an adaptable mindset and will soon find that you can train with, around, over or under, almost anything.

This, in turn, means that wherever you are, you can find some way to train. You may be a person who travels a lot for business and so is in a hotel room a lot of the time. Have a look round - is there a chair? You can use this to elevate your feet for push ups. You could also do reverse push ups, just sit with your back to the chair, place your hands on the seat and away you go.

Most times we have a wall close by! Let's look at some of the exercises we can do with the wall.

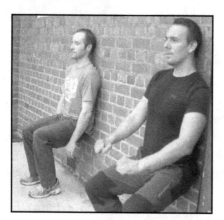

Use the wall as a support for a static squat. Keep the whole back flat against the wall and squat so the thighs are parallel to the floor.
Hold and keep the body as relaxed as possible, burst breath where needed.
This, or holding a chair in front, is a good way to practice squats if you have knee problems.

It allows you to keep good structure and so puts less pressure on the knees. As always, think safety first!

For a moving squat, try this. Stand with your back to the wall as before and go through your squat reps.

Now turn to the side and repeat, keeping contact to the wall with your foot, arm and hip. Turn face the wall and repeat. Then finish with reps on the opposite side as before.

For push-ups, use the feet to "climb" up the wall and practice inverted push-ups. From this position you can also "walk" along the wall if you have space.

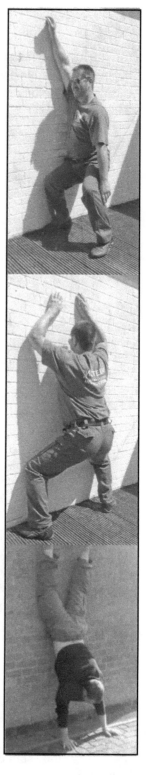

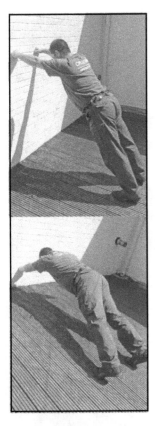

Try doing push-ups against the wall. Start from an upright position and gradually move your feet backwards.

If you can, go all the way to the floor then back up again.

You can use the wall to help with bridging exercises.

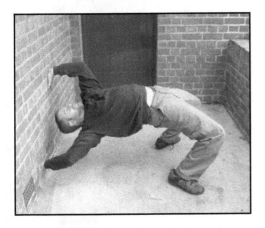

Stand with your back to the wall, place the palms back over your shoulders to the wall and then walk them down, slowly.

Another wall exercise is to stand facing the wall and fall forward into it. Bring the arms up, but collapse them rather than bracing yourself against the wall.

Once you have done this, as you impact the wall, roll out to the side, like you would with a side roll on the floor.

You can use the momentum to turn around and push yourself back off the wall.

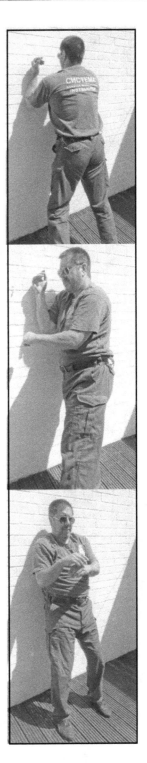

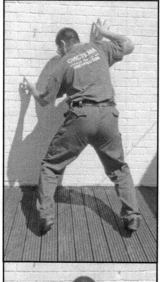

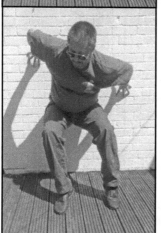

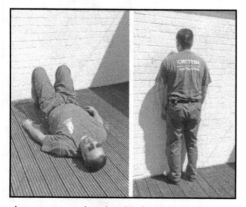

For finger strength, hold yourself against the wall with your fingertips and raise your heels.

Move around, always keeping the bodyweight on the fingers.

Change level, turn around and so on. Burst breath where necessary.

Lay on your back with legs bent feet on the floor and toes touching the wall. Stand up without moving the feet from their position.

Pull ups are another great upper body exercise. It may be difficult to have a proper pull up bar installed at your home, but there are plenty of other things we can use.

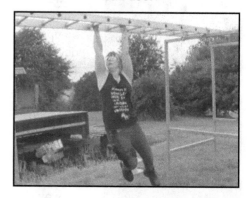

Suitable objects might include a strong beam, kids play equipment, a ladder secured between two points, even a tree branch. In each case, make sure the object is strong enough to support your weight and that you do not have too high a fall if you have to let go.

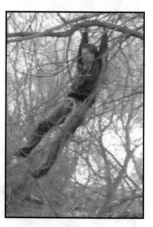

There are many variations on the standard pull up. You can vary the speed of course - try a 20 count. You can hang and raise the legs up to 90 degrees.

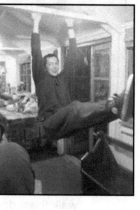

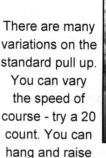

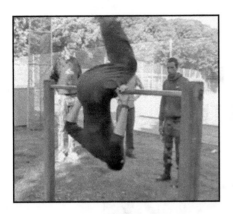

You can try lifting yourself, bringing the legs up and over, and rotating the body around the bar.

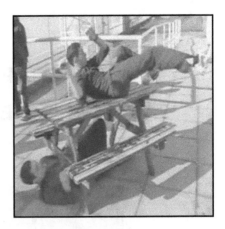

You can roll across and over picnic benches or gym benches, climb trees, go over, round or through any suitable object. Be sure to have permission to work in an area, and be aware of safety, particularly when climbing.

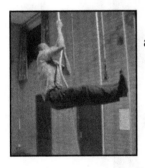

If you have access to an "old school" gym you may be able to practice climbing ropes, another great exercise.

Another option is to work on assault courses, if you can find one locally. If you can't find a "proper" assault course, have a look around and see what objects there are that you can use safely.

For an extra challenge, try working with your hands behind your back.

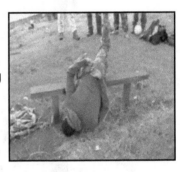

You may noticed I have not discussed the use of punchbags in this section. I have use them in the past but, to be honest, I have found them of little use in Systema training. You may get something from practicing basic strikes on a bag, if no partner is available, but it is much better to work with people to truly develop good striking skills.

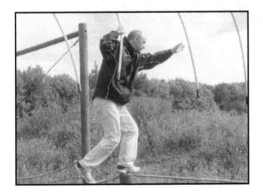

Many parks now have a "work out" space, see what is available in your area.

To sum up, be creative in your use of environment and equipment, learn to spot the opportunity in everything!

CHAPTER SIX

HEALTH

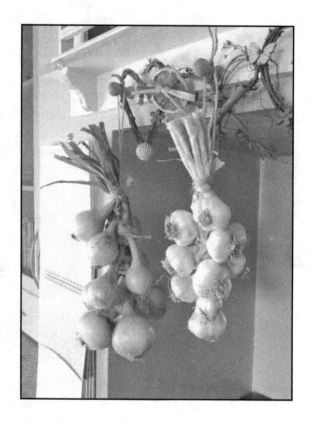

HEALTH

As we mentioned in the Introduction, health must be at the root of all our Systema training. It makes absolutely no sense, for people in a normal lifestyle to train in self defence and fitness in such a way that destroys their body.

I recently saw an on-line conversation between a group of martial artists who listed all their training injuries, as though they were badges of honour. They included broken bones, surgery, damaged joints, back problems and so on. You have to wonder if they would have sustained such severe injuries in having a few fights over the years! It is entirely possible to train well and hard without destroying the body in such a way. There is nothing "tough" about wrecking the most vital resource you have.

So, how do we approach solo health training from the Systema perspective? Once again we can think about the Four Pillars, this time as they relate to health - Movement, Massage, Diet and Mindset.

MOVEMENT

All the previous exercises we have looked at can be placed under this heading. Good, free movement is a vital aspect of our health and fitness regime. Unless monitored, over time our posture can collapse or become distorted. Even simple exercise helps remedy this and keeps the joints mobile and healthy. This, in turn, has a profound effect on our internal systems, in fact modern science is uncovering more and more connections between good, external exercises and our internal health and well being.

Movement also covers breathing of course and, if you can do nothing else at all, please at least put some regular breath work into your routine. You will find it has a marked effect on many aspects of your daily life

MASSAGE

If you think about it, massage is the oldest and most natural form of healing that we have. Bang your shin on a table and what is the first thing you do? Rub it, right?

There are many forms of massage treatment available but what, from a Systema perspective, can we do on our own? The first thing is to think of the ways we can massage ourselves. We can use different types of movement including; rubbing, kneading, tapping, friction, slapping, deep tissue, trigger point, washing and more, some using hands and some also possible with equipment.

The usual safety measures apply, particularly if you have an existing condition. Though it is difficult to cause yourself injury with light massage, always exercise care and caution. Breathing and posture are vital as always.

For "everyday" light massage you can work almost anywhere. For deeper massage work, find somewhere quiet and comfortable. You can use oils as required and it is good to practice some breathing with tension / relaxation prior to working. Let's start with some basic "muscle rubbing".

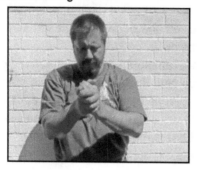

Begin by briskly rubbing the hands together to generate heat in the palms.

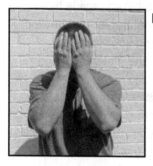

Keep the eyes open and cover them with the palms. Allow the heat from the hands to relax the muscles around the eyes. Hold for couple of minutes, then rub the hands together again.

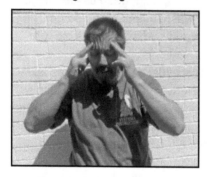

Using the palms and the fingers, work into all the muscle areas on the face. The pressure can be light, or heavier if there is a particular area of tension.

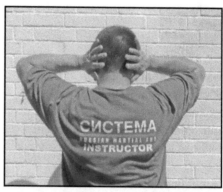

Work around the face, jaws and ears.

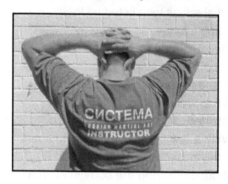

Link the fingers together and place the hands on the back of the head. Using the thumbs, press and stroke downwards into the neck muscles.

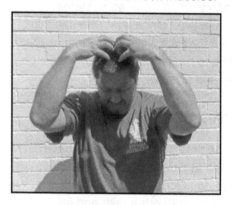

Tap the scalp gently with the fingertips. Start at the crown and work back, sideways and forward to cover the whole scalp.

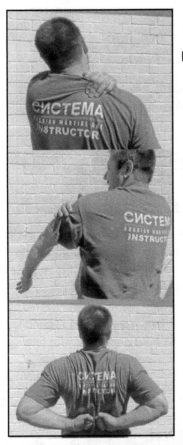

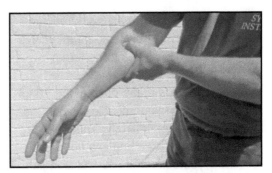

Use the same procedure and start working on the major muscle groups of the body. Rub gently at first.

Using the fists, rub into the lower back area, especially around the kidneys.

If you find an area that needs more work, then you can apply a deeper massage. One way to do this is with Trigger Point massage. You may feel that there is a knot or "lump" in the muscle at the sore point. Scientific opinion varies about the cause, but regardless, we can do something to ease the discomfort.

First, rub the point for about a minute. Now inhale and tense the muscle in question, hold for about 30 seconds. Exhale and relax the muscle. As you do so, press your finger / thumb directly into the knot. You can repeat this two or three times.

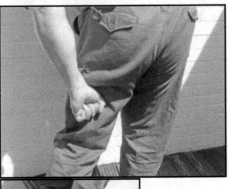

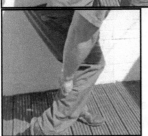

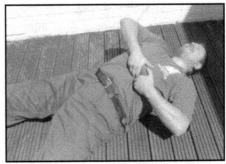

Continue this movement down into the legs. Rub into the thigh and calf muscles.

To massage around the torso, start under the ribs and work your fingers in as deep as you can. Exhale and relax as you push in. From the line of the ribs work down to cover the whole abdomen. This is very good for getting rid of deeper tension and is beneficial for the organs. If you find a sore spot, spend a little time working on it.

So that is basic rubbing or kneading massage, let us now look at percussive work. This takes three forms.

You can slap with the palm of the hand. Work all the major muscle groups and slap yourself quite firmly. This will bring blood to the area and is a good way "wake yourself up" if you feel sluggish.

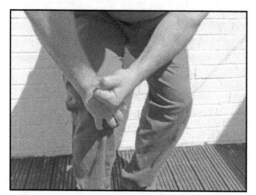

Tapping involves placing one hand on the body and using the other to "tap". For example, place one hand over the knee. Now form a fist with the other hand and firmly tap on the back of the first hand. You should feel the vibration go into the knee joint.

You can, of course, use the fist to "pummel" the muscles too. This can sometimes help a tense muscle to relax. Simply work all the major muscle groups as before.

EQUIPMENT

Almost anything can be used to assist with massage, particularly the equipment we discussed in the previous chapter. The knife handle, for example, can be used to work deeper into an area of tension. However, the two most useful items are the stick and the ball.

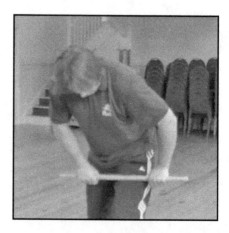

Use the stick to briskly rub the main muscle groups. Hold it in both hands and rub along the length of the muscle with the required amount of pressure.

You can even use a short stick to massage your own back with this procedure.

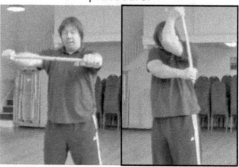

Hold the stick with both hands. Bring your right hand across and under the left, raise the left hand and reverse the grip.

Now take the left hand over your head and begin to move the stick down the back.

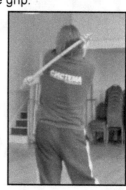

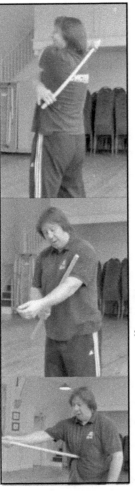

From here apply pressure with the stick and work into the back muscles. Simply move the hands up and down and pull.

The stick is also useful for percussive massage. Tap into the muscle groups as before. Hit lightly to stimulate the skin, or apply deeper hits into the muscle. Use the end of the stick to push into the muscle for deeper "point" massage.

size of a tennis or cricket ball is best. Simply roll the ball under the foot and put some weight into it. If you find a sore spot you can give it a little more pressure and attention.

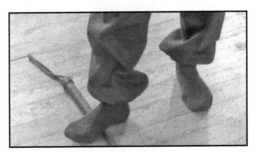

You can work the same massage with different object. There are specific "foot mats" available, I also like to use the Cossack whip. Roll the foot across it and walk along it's length.

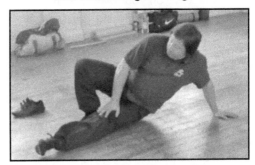

A ball is great for massaging the feet. We can gather a lot of tension in the feet and, whatever your views on reflexology, there is no doubt that a foot massage always makes us feel good!

I prefer to use a hard ball, it is actually a dog toy! About the

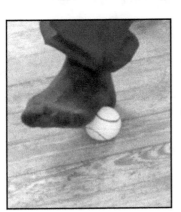

The ball can also be used for other parts of the body. Here, it is being rolled under the leg. Simply support yourself with one hand and let the body weight rest on the ball. Now slide yourself back and forth along the length of the muscle. You can do this for the legs, the back, the abdomen and so on. Again, a hard rubber ball is best for this work.

Foam rollers are becoming popular these days and they are a good tool for massage. You use them the same way you would a ball. Lay across the roller and slide along the muscle.

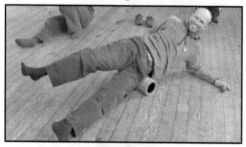

If you don't have a roller, you can work with a plastic drinks bottle. You need the 1 litre size, simply fill it with warm water and then use it as you would a roller.

Another aspect of massage is manipulation, or what you might call "chiropractic adjustment". This is a little difficult to do on your own, but there are

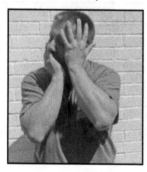

a couple of methods you can use.
To adjust the neck, place one hand under the chin, the other across the top of your head and push and pull sharply. Take care if you have an existing condition.

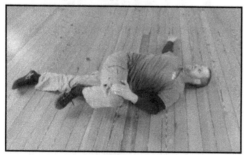

If you look back to our stretching exercises, you will find many of these postures are also useful for adjustments

- especially where we cross the knee over to one side. A sharp pull will often yield a satisfying "click" in the lower back!

These, then , are the basic methods of self massage. Take things easy at first, you can always build up intensity as required. If you find that a pain or discomfort is lingering, always get it checked out by your doctor or other qualified professional.

Of course you can use all these methods to massage another person. If you would like to try this, please be sure you are aware of any medical issues the person has prior to starting.

DIET

What we consume has an obvious affect on our health. We all know the dangers of too much sugar, processed foods, alcohol, tobacco and so on. There are many specific exercises out there and new ones that crop up all the time. Beware of falling for "fad" diets or whatever the "latest thing" is. Unless you have specific problems, the best nutritional advice I can think of is to prepare your own food as much as possible.

Try and avoid anything that is processed and stick to fresh fruit and vegetables. If you eat meat, try and source a local supplier rather than eat something that has been frozen who knows how many times and flown halfway around the world.

Personally I am always aware of issues of animal cruelty and prefer to avoid "industrialised meat" wherever possible. I have no scientific base for saying so, but have always felt that, moral questions aside, ingesting an animal that has had a horrible life and suffered unnecessary cruelty, may, on some level, have a detrimental effect on us.

Some, of course, choose to go vegetarian or vegan, on ethical, health and /or spiritual grounds. These are all things worthy of further research. The important thing is, whatever choice you make, to ensure a balanced diet and that your body is receiving all the correct amount of nutrients it needs to function properly. If there is a need to take supplements, once again do your research.

One way to ensure your food is fresh is to grow your own. You don't necessarily need a lot of space to grow some things, and a well-sized allotment or growing area allows you to grow a wide range of fruit and veg.

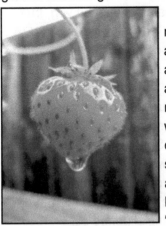

Numerous resources are available and you might also want to check to see if there are any local "growing groups" within your area.

Livestock is another possibility, though animals such as pigs and sheep are probably not practical for

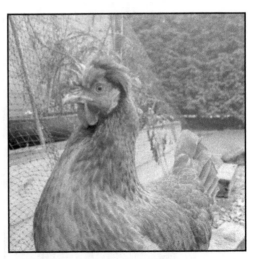

most of us, however, it doesn't take a lot of space to keep a few chickens. They are fairly low maintenance and will give you a daily supply of fresh eggs!

Bee-keeping is similarly rewarding and does not take a lot of space or time. Be sure to follow professional advice on setting up an apiary though!

FASTING

Fasting is an ancient practice, used in religious and health traditions around the world for thousands of years. . All animals do it occasionally, either by choice or by circumstance. By fasting, we mean taking a break from eating and drinking for 24-48 hours.

The first Western published research into fasting appeared in the late 19th century, since when thousands of studies have emerged, each finding fasting to have positive effects on obesity, cardiovascular disease, autoimmune disorders, diabetes, skin disease, gastrointestinal

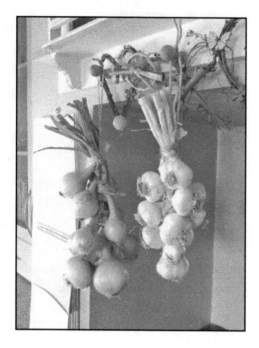

disease, arthritis and more. On a physical level, it is very good for the internal system to get a break. This gives the body a chance to remove toxins and eliminate weak and dying cells. On a psychological level, fasting helps strengthen self-control and can assist in weaning ourselves off of unhealthy foods or to start a new diet. There are three forms of fasting:

Dry Fasting - abstaining from all food and liquid.

Juice Fasting - abstaining from food and drink except water and pure vegetable and fruit juices.

Modified Fasting - eating only small amounts of food, usually raw fruit, and steamed veg, or drinking herbal teas or broths.

Fasting can last from one to three days and can be safely tolerated by most people. For periods longer than

this, or if you suffer from a medical condition, you should always consult a medical professional. We suggest a regular, weekly 24 hour fast as a good aid to health.

If you are fasting for the first time, try going without food for 12 or 18 hours to start and drink plenty of water. If you find that too hard, then try removing an ingredient out of your diet, for example meat or dairy products. Once you can do that, try a full 24 hour dry fast.

Where practical you should try and retain your daily routine, depending on workplace safety, of course. Don't boast or complain about your fast, one of the psychological aspects is to help you understand your limitations and teach you to deal with self-pity.

You can prepare for a fast by having a day of lighter eating to help your body adjust. Vegetarian meals are best, as animal products are harder to digest. So the day before you might try smaller meals of steamed veg, fruit and so on.

At the beginning of a fast you may experience hunger pains and slight headaches, but this should pass quickly. Your body may start ejecting toxins leading to a unpleasant taste in the mouth. Simply rinse your mouth with warm water.

When you fast, nonessential tissues, like fat, are used for fuel. During the initial period of conservation, the body functions with the same degree of efficiency and blood sugar levels remain fairly constant. After 24 hours, the body's metabolism can slow by as much as 75%, so for longer fasts be sure to include plenty of rest.

Once your fast is over, ease back into solid foods. Start with light meals, do not "binge" as this will place a heavy demand on your body and be counter productive.

So, to recap, start with a short fast and work up to 24 hours. Always check with your doctor prior to fasting, especially if you have an existing medical condition, are on prescription drugs and so on. Be aware of your activities during fasting and do nothing that may be dangerous if you become light headed.

Lastly, take the fasting process as an opportunity to review your overall diet and eating habits. Note, perhaps, how eating patterns are attached to certain emotional states and do your best to maintain a full, well balanced diet.

MINDSET

Our last, but by no means least, aspect of good personal health is mindset. This is a difficult quality to quantify, but what I mean is an overall positive aspect to life, rooted in personal beliefs and morality, but also prepared to be adaptable, creative and flexible. Aspirations and expectations must be tempered with reality. But likewise, we must be open to possibilities and opportunity.

If you regularly practice Systema breathing, exercises and so on, you should find it has a positive effect on

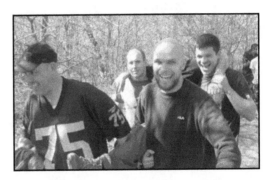

your mental outlook. The link between bodily activities and mental state has been long proven. Systema trains the practitioner to listen to their own body and explore their inner self . One aim of training is to familiarise an individual with their own body and psyche, become more in tune with how they feel and help understand their interactions with other people. So if good, regular exercise is a major component of a healthy mind, what are some others?

Family and friends give us a sense of belonging, of community and also a support network when times get hard. It is also good to make new friends, especially if you have perhaps moved to a new area, or find yourself in a more solitary situation. Get involved in your local community, take up a new hobby, go to see local sports, these are all easy ways of meeting and interacting with new people.

By the same token, we occasionally find people in our lives who exert a negative or even toxic influence. We have a choice when this happens - we can advise the person of their behaviour and help them adjust it., or we can work to exclude that person from our lives. This can be a difficult situation to deal with, but the important thing always is not to lose sight of our own positivity in the face of negative behaviour. Where family members are involved, or there are deeper problems, there are numerous agencies we can turn to for help.

Work can be a source of satisfaction, it can also be a source of stress, tension and worry. Aside from a lucky few, we all need to work in order to survive. If we are fortunate, we have a job that fulfils us in some way. More often, we take on a job simply as a way of paying our bills. I've worked in a range of jobs, from manual labour to clock watching in a sterile office and, with a few exceptions, didn't particularly enjoy any of it!

Work patterns are changing, so one thing to consider, if you hate your job, is can you change the conditions there? Could you work less hours and perhaps make the money up somewhere else? This may be another job or perhaps you can turn to a skill you have in order to generate income. Working for yourself is challenging and rewarding in equal measures, but it does give you the adaptability to manage your own time and work on different projects at once.

Work and money related stress is probably the single greatest cause of dis-ease in the developed world. It helps sometimes to put things into perspective. Consider how stressed you get when your train is late, compared to someone in another part of the world wondering if they will be able to feed their children today? Try to view any interruption to your daily routine as an opportunity. If you are sat on an immobile training for ten minutes, practice some breathing. Or, even more scary, chat to the people around you! Personal interaction is at an all time low, thanks to technology, and this can also have a profound affect on our mental well-being. Take your head out of your phone and interact with the world around you more!

Hobbies and activities provide us with an interest outside of ourselves. They may be creative, such as crafts, music, acting, or sports-related or you may enjoy travel, collecting, reading and so on. In each case, you hobby should give you a chance to interact with other people, to express yourself creatively or otherwise and to learn new skills and attributes.

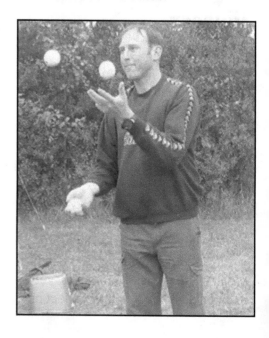

You are never too old to learn! If you find yourself getting a bit stagnant, take up juggling, enrol in an evening class for a new language, learn to play chess, join your local darts team, start horse-riding. Any and all of these things are possible without necessarily costing too much.

Another commendable activity is to volunteer for local services. This may be your local homeless shelter, or a national group such as the Samaritans. This way you also get to make a positive contribution to your community.

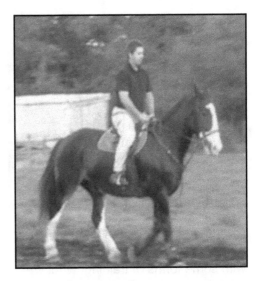

Reconnecting with nature is a great way to re-energise ourselves, particularly if you work indoors all the time. This can be as simple as taking a leisurely walk through your local park. Once again, put the phone away, take the time to take in the sights, sounds and smells around you.

If you have more time, take a day or two's break and head out into the wilds. It doesn't have to be the outback, a couple of days by the sea does wonders, or maybe some trekking through local forests. Of course all these locations give us great training opportunities too and my own group practices outdoors at least twice a month, whatever the weather.

If you would like to take this further, go on camping trips, or book up for an adventure holiday, a training camp or retreat. Learn how to make a fire, sleep out for a couple of nights. It will give you chance to get away from the normal routing and recharge your batteries.

Above all, the important thing is to have a measure of balance in your life between all your activities and also some sense of control. Nothing is more stressful than being in a situation that you have absolutely no control over. Now, to be honest, that covers just about everything! Even just recognising and dealing with that fact helps ease stress. After all, if we can't control it, then what is the point of stressing over it? Instead, we look to what elements in a situation we can

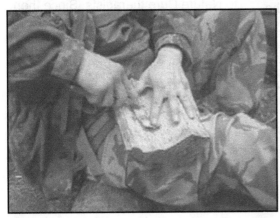

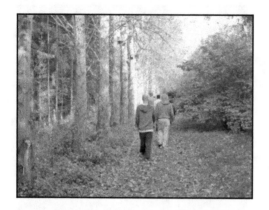

control and work to address them in a positive way. This is where I take issue with some forms of training, what we might call the "what if?" school of thought. This is where there is a specific tool or technique for every conceivable situation. Aside from issues of the thought-process behind selecting the correct technique within a second of something happening, it ignores another fundamental truth. That is that the one constant in *everything* that happens to you, in *every* situation you are in, wherever you are….is *you*.

If this is the one constant, it surely makes sense to understand and know how to best "operate" yourself in stressful conditions. This is why breathing and "internal work" is at the heart of all good Systema training. External movement, fine or gross motor skills, split second judgement calls are nothing without that particular internal state that we aim for.

There are several well laid out paths we can follow to develop our "internal monitor" and they all begin with basic breathing exercises. So, whatever else you do in terms of

physical exercise, please look into the Systema breathing methods, as put forward by Mikhail and Vladimir, and put them to use in your life. The deeper you go with them, the more profound and beneficial effects you will discover.

ENERGY WORK

There is one more area of health training I'd like to discuss and that is "energy work". I am keeping the term "energy" rather vague and for a purpose. This term always seems to provoke strong reactions in martial art circles, perhaps due to some of the dubious "empty force" clips that regularly do the rounds.

That aside, if we look at the medical / spiritual background of many cultures, it is not uncommon to find reference to "energy". It forms the base of traditional Chinese medical theory and its system of acupuncture, qigong for example.

From a Western perspective, the concept of a human energy field in natural medicine goes back 200 years to Nature Cure therapists. Since then there have been numerous studies on the body's "energy field", with various results and, of course, widely differing opinions.

If this all seems a little vague, then think of it in these terms. Those previous health methods we discussed – movement, diet, breathing, mindset – all give a certain energy to the body. Movement produces energy, food gives us nutrients, breathing gives us oxygen and our mindset is responsible for directing and monitoring it all. There can be little doubt that mindset is a factor in health.

Think, then, of combining all these elements and using the mindset to "direct" the energy. But you don't have to think it, you can try this simple exercise and feel for yourself.

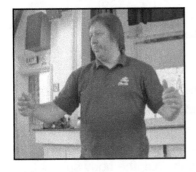

Find a quiet spot, sit or stand in a comfort able position. We are doing two movements, allied to breathing. On an inhale, we take the hands apart, out to the sides. On an

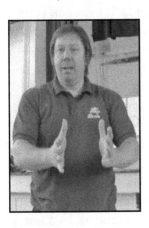

exhale we bring the hands together until the palms are almost touching. The arms should be relaxed. But maintain a slight tension in the palms. As you open, relax the hands a little and let the palms close. As you bring the hands together, the fingers stretch and the hands open out, as though you are pushing from the centre of the palm.

That's the physical component. Now, as the palms come together, imagine a slight force is keeping them apart, just like when you push two magnet of the same pole together.

Allow your breathing to slow, focus on nothing else but the breathing and the hands. After a while you may feel a sensation in the hands, a heat, or a tingling, or something else. Let this develop for a while. Once you have that feeling, you can begin rolling the hands around, as though holding a ball between them and see if the feeling strengthens.

Once the feeling is strong, do the head and face massage we showed before, but this time with very light or no contact. Keep the palms about an inch away from the skin. If this is successful you can do similar work over any other part of the body, particularly any spot where you have an injury or problem.

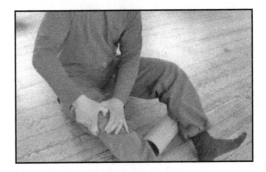

So what is it that we are feeling? Is it pure imagination? Maybe, but as many placebo trials and other tests have shown, the imagination can have a powerful effect on the body. Is it an "energy field", or something similar? That is for you to decide, there is plenty of information and opinion, scientific and otherwise, out there on the Internet. The important thing is that you try the method and see what results you get.

There is another very powerful exercise for our overall health and "energetic" well-being, and that is cold water dousing. This has received more and more attention over recent years, but has been practiced in some cultures since ancient times. The easiest and most effective method I have found is to simply to pour over the head water from one or two large buckets whilst standing barefoot outside.

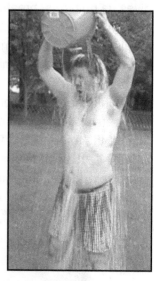

burst breath a little, especially if you are out in cold weather. It is good to do this practice on a regular basis, once or even twice a day if you have time. A cold shower is a substitute when you can't get outside, but I've found is not quite the same effect.

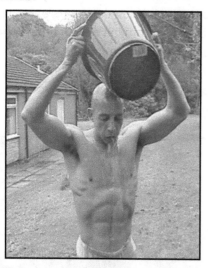

Prepare your bucket before hand and it is good to let it stand for a while. If the weather is quite warm, you might want to add some ice to the bucket so the water really is cold! Stand in a comfortable position and inhale. Raise the bucket and slowly and smoothly pour the water over the crown of your head, as you exhale. Following this,

So what does this dousing do? In response to cold, the body shoots up its core temperature to over 40 degrees, which kills off most viruses and bacteria. It stimulates many of the body systems and will increase your resistance to cold. From an "energy" perspective, some claim it cleanses the energy field and helps us "reconnect" with the earth (hence being barefoot). Overall, it will wake you up and give you a warm glow and will also strengthen you psychologically in much the same way that fasting does.

The hardest step is the first, but just set your mind and give it a try. Once you have experienced it a few times you will want to do it every day! Just remember, balance in all things.

Another aspect of "internal" work is the idea of prayer, meditation or contemplation. If you are a religious person I'll presume that you already have some experience of prayer and contemplation. For Christians, the Jesus Prayer is a particularly useful method. If you are not religious but would like to discover more, I advise talking to a suitably qualified person at your local temple, church or mosque. If you are not religious and are not interested in religion, but would like to practice "meditation", I advise the following simple routine.

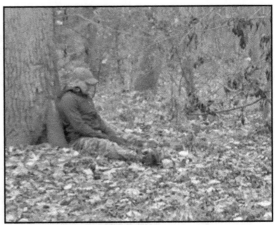

Set aside a quiet place and time. Make sure you will not be interrupted, so turn off your phone! Sit in a comfortable position; don't worry about being in a particular posture. Your hands can rest in your lap, or you can use the hand movement we described earlier. Keep the back straight and begin breathing. Use the square pattern, so begin by counting two on and inhale, two on an exhale. Work your way up to ten then back down. Then find a number you are comfortable with and stick with that.

As you breathe in, imagine the air filling the lungs and body with clean, pure energy. As you exhale, imagine the lungs and body releasing all the toxins with the out breath.

Mentally, focus only on the breathing and posture. If and when your thoughts wander, let them come and go, don't attach to them, bring your mind back to the breath. Try this for five or ten minutes and I think you will find it mentally "refreshing". You can build up the time, of course, though 15

or 20 minutes is long enough. When you finish, bring your focus back to your surroundings and sit quietly for another minute. Then stand slowly and do a few gentle exercises to get the body moving again.

There are deeper methods of meditation, some of which I studied in depth for many years. Personally, they are something I have moved away from, in favour of prayer, but it is up to each of us to find their own path. If nothing else, at least find some "quiet time" in your life where all you have to do is "sit and be" for a while.

A final word on health practices – be open to new ideas but always be aware of medical issues and avoid extremes. Anything that may bring harm to the body or you think may be damaging psychologically should be questioned. Be wary of any person or group who attempts to exert psychological control over you through their methods. Such a situation is far from healthy. In short, move, breathe, eat well and enjoy your life!

CHAPTER SEVEN
PROGRESSION

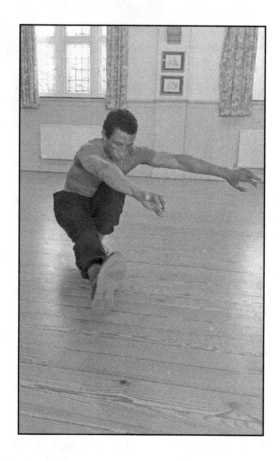

PROGRESSION

The previous chapters cover many of the basic methods of solo training and, if you are new to Systema, should give you a solid foundation. But where do you go from there? If you are part of a training group or club, I'm sure your Instructor will be showing you new ideas and exercises all the time. If you train on your own, though, or are looking for some ways to advance your work, here are some ideas. Let's start with some variations on the Core Exercises.

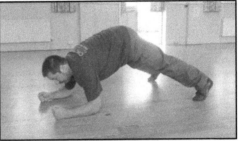

From the normal push up position rotate the fists back to support yourself on the forearms, then rotate forward to return to the start position.

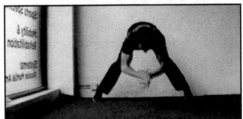

Push up and clap on the lift. You can try hand claps under the body, out to the front or, for a real challenge, behind your back.

Once you can do the push up comfortably, try doing the exercise on one hand.

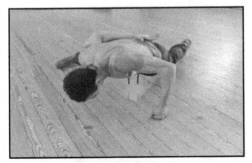

You can bring the feet wider apart to help.

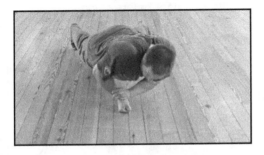

Or hold the supporting forearm with your free hand for support.

Do a palm push up and as you raise up, turn and stretch one hand as high as you can. Bring the hand back to the floor for the down move, then repeat on the other side.

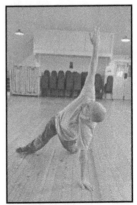

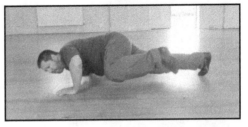

From palm press up position, each time you lower bring the knee up towards the elbow. Repeat on each side.

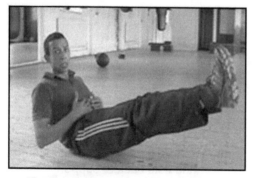

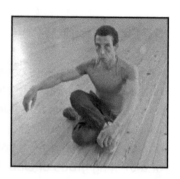

Go all the way to the floor, then twist and rise to the start position.

If you want to make the sit up more challenging, try lifting the body and feet at the same time. You can also work on holding this as a static position.

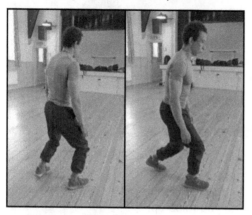

One squat variation is the spiral squat.

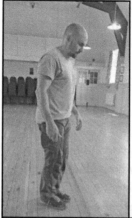

Another squat variation is to take one leg back.

Start in normal position. As you lower, bring your arms forward for balance and take one foot back.

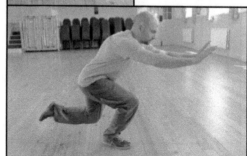

Start from normal position, then shift your weight into one leg.

Allow the rear heel to lift as you turn and sink.

Slowly squat down, keeping the back straight and the body relaxed.

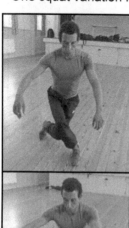

If you can, go all the way to the floor before rising.

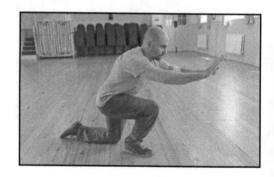

A squat where you take one leg forward is called a pistol squat. This is a challenging exercise and should only be attempted once you can do a normal squat smoothly with correct form.
It is best to practice step by step.
Try at first going into a low squat position and simply shift as much weight as you can from leg to leg.

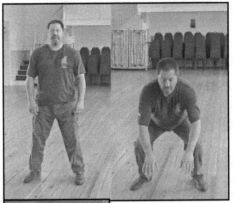

Following this, use a suitable object (or person!) for support. Slowly lower down on one leg as far as you are comfortable. If your posture starts changing to compensate, rise back up. Step by step you will eventually be able to go to the floor supported. Then repeat the process with no support.

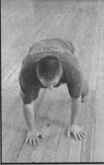

When you are proficient at pistol squats and want an even greater challenge, try working on a wobble board. Always take great care with this exercise, be sure to maintain good knee/foot alignment and remember to breathe!

You can use the squat as a method to get to the floor. Start in normal position, squat and bring your hands to the ground.

Keep the arms

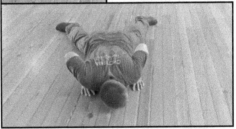

relaxed to absorb the force as you come the ground and slide your feet back.

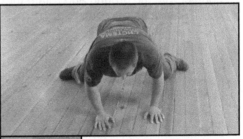

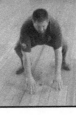

To get back up, pull your hips forward and up into a squat, then stand. You can do this slow, or fast, like a burpee.

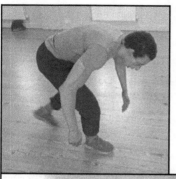

Another "standing to floor" exercise is the modified sprawl.

Take one foot back

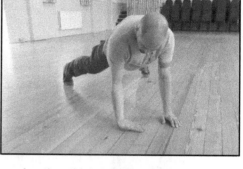

Another thing to think about is how different types of exercise can be combined. Here, for example, we add joint rotation into a push up.
Work on the palms and rotate one hand out. You can keep the hand in place

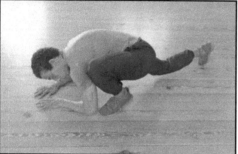

and drop forward to the ground. Support yourself on forearms and toes.

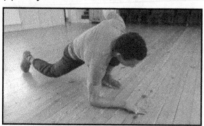

You can use the same movement to get to the floor and roll. Get three points of contact with the ground and rotate the support arm outward.

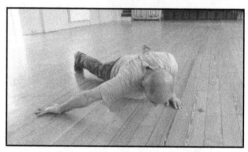

or use the rotation to slide the arm out to the side as you lower down.

Using this method you can add shoulder rolls into squats, chest rotation into sit ups and many other variations.

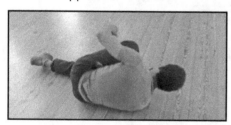

Follow the rotation of the arm to bring the shoulder and body to the floor and roll out to the side.

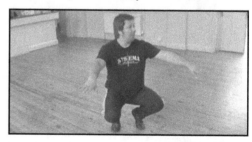

In short, once you have a good grasp of the basic core exercise, work to add in as many variations as you can, in posture, speed, breathing pattern and levels of tension. Then see how you can add in extra body movements.

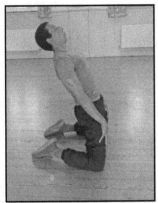

The same principle applies to stretching. Once you are comfortable with the basic movements, you can try more challenging positions.

From a seated position, swing your legs back behind you and fall forward onto your torso.

Try not to use your hands, but arch the body back slightly and turn the head to

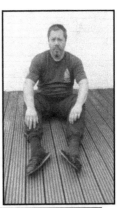

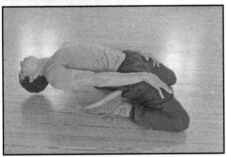

Get into a kneeling position and slowly bend back. Work to keep the thighs are relaxed as possible. If necessary, hold at your "stop point" and burst breathe to help relax the muscles.

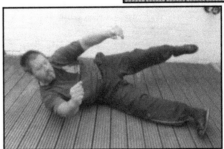

the side. Exhale as you fall.

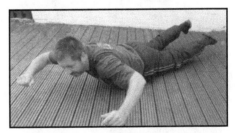

From there, swing your legs back round to the start position

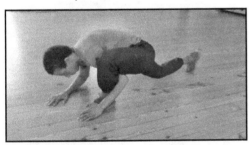

Also explore how you can use the exercise positions themselves in order to stretch. Here we see the modified squat being held as a static stretch posture.

Now let's look at some other methods of falling. As always, be aware of safety issues and make sure you are able to fall comfortably from "normal" positions before trying the more advanced falls. It's perfectly fine to train on mats to start with.

To practice sideways falling, start in a sitting position.

Allow the body to fall to the side and extend an arm out.

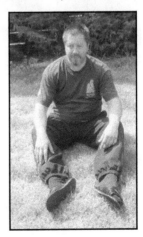

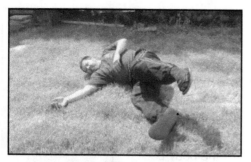

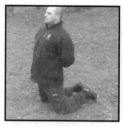

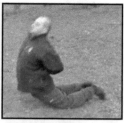

Get into kneeling position and place the hands behind the back. Arch the body forward and let yourself fall.

As the hand contacts the floor, allow it to slide away, so bringing the body smoothly to the ground. Relax and exhale on the fall.

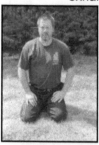

Now repeat the same procedure from a kneeling position.

Let the hand slide again, do not brace the arm.

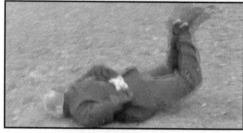

Once again, exhale, turn the head to the side and make sure the body is arched so the impact is absorbed by the "rocking" of the body.

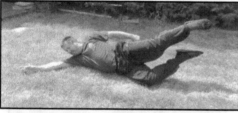

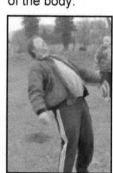

From normal standing position, lean back until you feel your balance start to go.

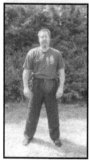

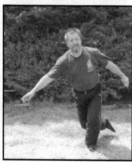

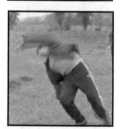

Let yourself fall and, as you go, turn the body and sweep one arm up and around in front of you.

Finally work from standing. To fall, you can take one leg back behind the other and fall as before.

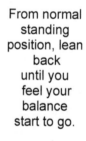

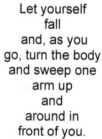

Let the arm contact the floor as you fall into a forward roll.

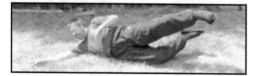

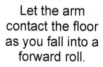

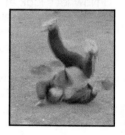

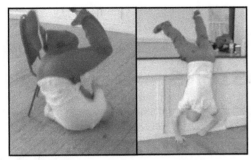

Once you are comfortable working over chairs, try going from a greater height. Go slow to start, always be sure to protect the head from impact, exhale and relax the body.

We mentioned earlier that there are many great resources available from Systema HQ on breathing that we highly recommend.
However I will add in one more breathing exercise here, as it is very good for developing muscle control, learning to move tension and is a gateway exercise to deeper, internal work.

We are going to take a long inhale, then an equal exhale.

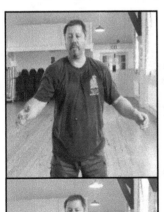

Next relax the upper arm and tense the shoulder/chest. This completes the inhale.

On the exhale, follow the same procedure down to the opposite fist.

So the tension moves through

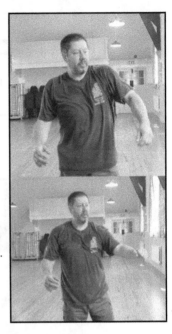

As we breathe, we move a "ball of tension" from one hand to the other.

So, as the inhale starts, tense the fist. As the inhale continues, relax the fist and tense the forearm.

Relax the forearm and tense the upper arm.

the shoulder/chest, into the upper arm, the forearm and then the fist. Finally the fist relaxes as the exhale ends.

Practice this a few times, then reverse the movement back the other way (so if you began by tensing the left fist, now start with the right). Once you have the idea, try the same exercise with the tension moving from foot to foot, each way.
From here, try linking different parts of the body and moving the tension between them with the breath.

As you progress, the outward movement of tension should become less and less visible. Discover how you tense "internally" by manipulating not just the muscles but also the tendons and the nervous system.

This simple, but deep, exercise brings many benefits. Any tension that comes into the body can easily be shifted away. Not just physical tension, but also psychological tension and fear. If you can move the tension you can also "recycle" it into a strike or similar.

CHAPTER EIGHT
CONCLUSIONS

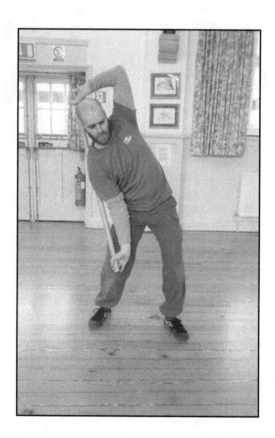

CONCLUSIONS

I hope the previous chapters give you some good ideas on solo training and also a pointer for future development. As mentioned at the start, it would be impossible to include every single solo exercise in one book, so bear in mind what you see here is just the tip of the iceberg! The question now is, how do you arrange all this information and fit it into your schedule? I don't know how long it would take to go through every exercise in this book, but I'm guessing it would be hours, and most of us do not have that kind of time available on a daily basis.

There are two methods to organising your solo training. The first is to create a schedule. So let's say you have half an hour each day that you can put aside for training. Get a notebook and draw up a schedule for each day. You can focus on different things on specific days. For example, your Monday session may be mostly stretching, breathing and core exercises. Tuesday is about ground mobility. Wednesday you go for a run, and so on. You start with the basics and, over time, increase the challenge level of each exercise.

This method gives you a nice clear structure and you can also set yourself targets, eg *by June I aim to be doing 20 push ups with a breath hold.*

This is a good approach to take if you are new to training / Systema. It allows you to focus on those areas that need the most work, while still getting a good overall coverage of exercise types. Of course the amount of time you have each day may vary, so you can adjust accordingly. The important thing is to be consistent, not do nothing for four days then try and cram everything into one session on Thursday.

The second method is to be more fluid in your approach, fit your exercise in where you can throughout the day. This is the approach I favour at the moment, partly due to having a reasonable base in the fundamentals and also having an irregular work pattern.

So if you find you have ten minutes spare, do some exercise. If you take the dog for a walk, use the chance to get some jogging and square breathing in. The downside to this approach is you need to make

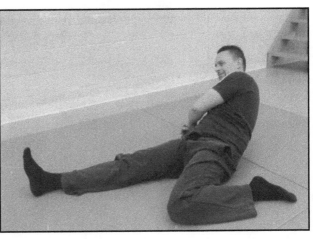

sure you take the opportunities to exercise and not think "I'll have a cup of tea instead".

I'd also still recommend you set aside a couple of longer sessions once or twice a week where you can. It is also important to vary the intensity of your session. This is not about driving yourself hard into the ground at every available opportunity, nor is it about being "easy" on yourself. The aim is to get a good overall balance in your exercise regime. Balance strength training with mobility, speed with relaxation, above all always deal with any extra stress brought into your system with breathing and massage.

Speaking of balance, there is nothing wrong with taking a day off now and then. Don't become obsessed and let exercise take over or get in the way of family life! If you are training for a specific event, of course, you can adjust according to the needs of that event. But after, get back into your regular routine.

One other thing, please don't post what you are doing up on social media! I know a guy who used to this, every day he would post "just done 40 push ups!". No one cares and it smacks of attention seeking or a need to be noticed and acknowledged in some way.

Excessive physical exercise, or other activities, are often symptomatic of an underlying psychological issue (think of certain dietary disorders for example, or Body Dismorphia). Best to have the underlying issue looked at and dealt with by a professional before you potentially damage yourself further through your physical actions. Always be sure to check with your Dr prior to exercising if you have a medical condition and if any exercises causes you pain or distress, stop it immediately!

Please take on board what we have said about adapting and creating exercises for your own needs and, of course, many Systema Instructors and others put lots of good ideas out on social media.

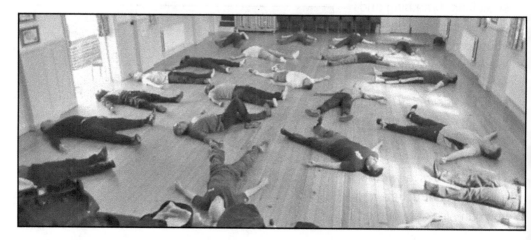

Think about how you can combine exercises from across the different chapters – so you could, for example, combine getting up and down from the floor with the sledgehammer. You can go into dives and rolls while running. And, of course, you can and should apply breathing to everything. I hope this will go some way to changing your mindset from "exercise" to "activity". You will then understand how "exercise" can actually be part of your everyday activities. If you can grasp this, you can be training all the time!

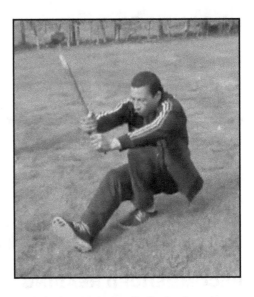

I want to leave you with one last concept and it pertains to what Systema "is", or at least one way it can be viewed. Human beings consist of the following:

1. Nervous System
2. Cardiovascular System
3. Respiratory System
4. Genito-urinary System
5. Digestive System
6. Lymphatic/immune System
7. Muscular-skeletal System

In addition we might be said to possess physical, psychological and spiritual aspects to our make up. Training in Systema is designed to work on and through each and every one of these systems. Frequently an exercise might work on several systems at once. Even a simple push-up, performed in a particular way with certain breathing patterns can be working on the respiratory, muscular and psychological systems simultaneously.

Systema is designed to bring you personally an awareness of all of these systems and their strengths and weaknesses. So one way to approach your solo work is to think what "systems" you would like to train and adapt your exercise accordingly.

As Vladimir describes, this is also why Systema can be called *poznai sebia* or *Know Yourself*. This, on all sorts of levels, promotes our understanding of ourselves and others. If you can truly understand yourself and others, self defence, survival, in fact life in general, takes on a whole different perspective. Doing what is necessary in any situation becomes clearer. Understanding destroys the two biggest killers – fear (stress) and ego (pride).

Good luck in your training!

RESOURCES

Mikhail Ryabko
Systema HQ Moscow   www.systemaryabko.com

Vladimir Vasiliev
Systema HQ Toronto   www.russianmartialart.com

Robert Poyton
Cutting Edge Systema   www.systemauk.com

Books and Downloads   www.systemafilms.com

RECOMMENDED READING

Strikes - Vladimir Vasiliev & Scott Meredith

Let Every Breath - Vladimir Vasiliev

The Systema Manual - Major Konstantin Komarov

The Ten Points of Sparring   - Robert Poyton

Systema Partner Training - Robert Poyton

Systema Awareness   - Robert Poyton

Systema Locks, Holds & Throws   - Robert Poyton

Systema Voices   - -ed. Robert Poyton

NOTES

Printed in the USA
CPSIA information can be obtained
at www.ICGtesting.com
LVHW080727260923
759260LV00006B/919

9 780995 645431